AF892407

Neurorehabilitation and Physical Therapy

Edited by Hideki Nakano

Published in London, United Kingdom

Neurorehabilitation and Physical Therapy
http://dx.doi.org/10.5772/intechopen.102185
Edited by Hideki Nakano

Contributors
Hideki Nakano, Ryu Ushio, Kousuke Tamura, Shoya Fujikawa, Chihiro Ohsumi, Shun Sawai, Ryosuke Yamamoto, Joseph Nshimiyimana, Jean Claude Muhigirwa, Potien Uwihoreye, Theogene Niyonsenga, Monika Šorfová, Jaroslav Langer, David Ravnik, Ashna Sinha, Meena Gupta, Andrés J. Ursa Herguedas, Emilio J. Guzón González, Elzbieta Trylinska-Tekielska, Dorota Pietraszewska, Iwona Stanisłąwska, Ada Holak, Biraj Bhattarai, Hema Nagaraj

© The Editor(s) and the Author(s) 2023
The rights of the editor(s) and the author(s) have been asserted in accordance with the Copyright, Designs and Patents Act 1988. All rights to the book as a whole are reserved by INTECHOPEN LIMITED. The book as a whole (compilation) cannot be reproduced, distributed or used for commercial or non-commercial purposes without INTECHOPEN LIMITED's written permission. Enquiries concerning the use of the book should be directed to INTECHOPEN LIMITED rights and permissions department (permissions@intechopen.com).
Violations are liable to prosecution under the governing Copyright Law.

Individual chapters of this publication are distributed under the terms of the Creative Commons Attribution 3.0 Unported License which permits commercial use, distribution and reproduction of the individual chapters, provided the original author(s) and source publication are appropriately acknowledged. If so indicated, certain images may not be included under the Creative Commons license. In such cases users will need to obtain permission from the license holder to reproduce the material. More details and guidelines concerning content reuse and adaptation can be found at http://www.intechopen.com/copyright-policy.html.

Notice
Statements and opinions expressed in the chapters are these of the individual contributors and not necessarily those of the editors or publisher. No responsibility is accepted for the accuracy of information contained in the published chapters. The publisher assumes no responsibility for any damage or injury to persons or property arising out of the use of any materials, instructions, methods or ideas contained in the book.

First published in London, United Kingdom, 2023 by IntechOpen
IntechOpen is the global imprint of INTECHOPEN LIMITED, registered in England and Wales, registration number: 11086078, 5 Princes Gate Court, London, SW7 2QJ, United Kingdom

British Library Cataloguing-in-Publication Data
A catalogue record for this book is available from the British Library

Additional hard and PDF copies can be obtained from orders@intechopen.com

Neurorehabilitation and Physical Therapy
Edited by Hideki Nakano
p. cm.
Print ISBN 978-1-80356-344-2
Online ISBN 978-1-80356-345-9
eBook (PDF) ISBN 978-1-80356-346-6

We are IntechOpen, the world's leading publisher of Open Access books
Built by scientists, for scientists

6,200+
Open access books available

168,000+
International authors and editors

185M+
Downloads

156
Countries delivered to

Our authors are among the
Top 1%
most cited scientists

12.2%
Contributors from top 500 universities

WEB OF SCIENCE™

Selection of our books indexed in the Book Citation Index in Web of Science™ Core Collection (BKCI)

Interested in publishing with us?
Contact book.department@intechopen.com

Numbers displayed above are based on latest data collected.
For more information visit www.intechopen.com

Meet the editor

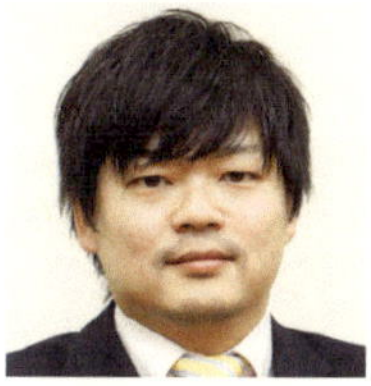

Dr. Hideki Nakano is a physical therapist and associate professor at the Neurorehabilitation Laboratory, Graduate School of Health Sciences, Kyoto Tachibana University, Japan. He received his Ph.D. in Health Science from Kio University, Japan, and has accepted research training experience as a JSPS Research Fellow at Neurorehabilitation Research Center, Kio University, Japan, and Queensland Brain Institute, The University of Queensland, Australia. He specializes in neuroscience, neurophysiology, and rehabilitation science and conducts research using non-invasive brain function measurement and brain stimulation methods such as electroencephalography, transcranial magnetic stimulation, and transcranial electrical stimulation. His current main research interest is developing rehabilitation evaluation and treatment methods using visualization and manipulation methods of brain functions for healthy, elderly, and diseased patients.

Contents

Preface **IX**

Section 1
Basic Research **1**

Chapter 1 **3**
Application of Attention Focus in Rehabilitation to Promote Motor Performance and Motor Learning
by Shun Sawai, Shoya Fujikawa, Ryosuke Yamamoto and Hideki Nakano

Chapter 2 **27**
Potential Applications of Motor Imagery for Improving Standing Posture Balance in Rehabilitation
by Shoya Fujikawa, Chihiro Ohsumi, Ryu Ushio, Kousuke Tamura, Shun Sawai, Ryosuke Yamamoto and Hideki Nakano

Chapter 3 **43**
Clinical Application of Repetitive Peripheral Magnetic Stimulation in Rehabilitation
by Ryu Ushio, Kousuke Tamura, Shoya Fujikawa, Chihiro Ohsumi, Shun Sawai, Ryosuke Yamamoto and Hideki Nakano

Chapter 4 **55**
Possibility of Using a VR System as an Action Observation Therapeutical Technique
by Jaroslav Langer, Monika Šorfová and David Ravnik

Section 2
Clinical Research **65**

Chapter 5 **67**
Effect of Unilateral Neglect with Basal Ganglia Bleed in Stroke Survivor
by Ashna Sinha and Meena Gupta

Chapter 6 **79**
Neurofunctional Intervention Approaches
by Joseph Nshimiyimana, Potien Uwihoreye, Jean Claude Muhigirwa and Theogene Niyonsega

Chapter 7 **105**
Nutritional Support in Stroke Neurorehabilitation
by Andrés J. Ursa Herguedas and Emilio J. Guzón González

Chapter 8 **117**
Mild Cognitive Impairment: An Overview
by Biraj Bhattarai and Hema Nagaraj

Chapter 9 **131**
Methods of Treating Autism: Holistic Approach to the Rehabilitation of People with the Spectrum of Autism
by Elzbieta Trylinska-Tekielska, Dorota Pietraszewska, Iwona Stanisawska and Ada Holak

Preface

In recent years, neurorehabilitation (neuroscience-based rehabilitation), which utilizes the brain's plasticity, has made remarkable progress and attracted much attention. The term "neurorehabilitation" is defined as "concepts, evaluation methods, therapies, and devices that apply the knowledge of brain theory revealed by neuroscience and related research to rehabilitation medicine." The concept of neurorehabilitation is widely accepted in physical therapy, and evaluation and treatment based on this concept are being practiced. What is required in neurorehabilitation research is to analyze the changes and improvements in motor behavior and cognitive and learning abilities and the changes in brain functions that bring about these changes. This will allow us to get closer to the neural mechanisms of rehabilitation effects and is expected to develop effective methods that are more suitable for the subject. The book presents basic research and clinical applications related to neurorehabilitation and physical therapy. It is organized into the following nine chapters written by experts from around the world.

Chapter 1: "Application of Attention Focus in Rehabilitation to Promote Motor Performance and Motor Learning"

Chapter 2: "Potential Applications of Motor Imagery for Improving Standing Posture Balance in Rehabilitation"

Chapter 3: "Clinical Application of Repetitive Peripheral Magnetic Stimulation in Rehabilitation"

Chapter 4: "Possibility of Using a VR System as an Action Observation Therapeutical Technique"

Chapter 5: "Effect of Unilateral Neglect with Basal Ganglia Bleed in Stroke Survivor"

Chapter 6: "Neurofunctional Intervention Approaches"

Chapter 7: "Nutritional Support in Stroke Neurorehabilitation"

Chapter 8: "Mild Cognitive Impairment: An Overview"

Chapter 9: "Methods of Treating Autism: Holistic Approach to the Rehabilitation of People with the Spectrum of Autism"

I would like to express my great appreciation to the authors of this book and all those involved in its editing.

Hideki Nakano, Ph.D.
Associate Professor,
Neurorehabilitation Laboratory,
Graduate School of Health Sciences,
Kyoto Tachibana University,
Kyoto, Japan

Section 1

Basic Research

Chapter 1

Application of Attention Focus in Rehabilitation to Promote Motor Performance and Motor Learning

Shun Sawai, Shoya Fujikawa, Ryosuke Yamamoto and Hideki Nakano

Abstract

Attention focus plays an essential role in promoting motor performance and motor learning. There are two types of attention focus: internal focus and external focus. Internal focus refers to direct attention inside the body while external focus refers to direct attention outside the body. Several studies have reported that external focus positively affects motor performance and motor learning by promoting automatic control. The mechanisms of attention focus have been examined using electromyography (EMG), electroencephalography (EEG), and functional magnetic resonance imaging (fMRI). During rehabilitation, therapists promote patients' movement acquisition and motor learning. This chapter reviews the application of attention focus in rehabilitation to promote motor performance and motor learning in patients.

Keywords: attention focus, internal focus, external focus, performance, motor learning, rehabilitation

1. Introduction

When a person exercises, their attention is somewhere else. Attention focus describes a change in behavior depending on the focus of one's attention. Attention focus can be divided into internal focus and external focus. Internal focus is defined as "instructions related to the learner's own body movements." External focus is defined as "instructions related to the effects of the performer's actions on the environment, for example, the experimental apparatus" [1]. Several studies have reported that external focus is more effective for performance and motor learning than internal focus. The positive effects of external focus are explained by the constrained action hypothesis (CAH). The CAH states that "trying to consciously control one's movements constrains the motor system by interfering with automatic motor control processes that would "normally" regulate the movement" [2]. Based on the CAH, internal focus promotes conscious control of movement by directing attention to inside the body, inhibiting the automatic control of movement, resulting in a negative effect. In contrast, external focus positively inhibits conscious control of movements and promotes automatic control of movements by directing the individual's attention externally. In this chapter, the effects of internal focus and external focus on changes in performance and motor learning are summarized. In addition, the application of attention focus in the field of rehabilitation is discussed.

1.1 The origin of attention focus

The first study regarding attention focus was reported by Wulf et al. [1] who examined the effects of internal focus and external focus on motor learning during a slalom movement using a ski simulator. The participants moved rhythmically to the left and right with as wide amplitude as possible. The study was divided into three groups: internal focus, external focus, and a control group who did not receive instructions regarding attention focus. Participants in the internal focus group were instructed to "try to exert force on the outer foot." Participants in the external focus group were instructed to "try to exert force on the outer wheels as long as the platform moved in the respective direction." Therefore, the attention of the participants in the internal focus group was directed to their feet and that in the external focus group was directed to the ski simulator. The amplitude of the movements increased with task performance, and greater learning retention was observed in the external focus group than in the internal focus and control groups. The task performance was the worst in the internal focus group. Although changes in performance due to attention had been examined previously, the classification of attention focus as internal focus and external focus led to the development of studies regarding attention focus. This inaugural study also reported the positive effects of paying attention to the outside of the body (external focus) and the negative effects of paying attention to the inside of the body (internal focus). Subsequently, the effects of attention focus during various tasks have been examined.

1.2 Attention focus during balance control and sports activities

The effects of attention focus on healthy participants have been examined during several tasks that require accuracy, including balance tasks and sports activities. Several studies have examined the effects of attention focus on performance and motor learning during center of pressure sway (COP) control using a stabilometer. As it is difficult to observe the effect of attention focus during simple tasks [3], studies that include healthy young participants often include difficult postural tasks or tasks performed on rough surfaces. For example, previously-used tasks include posture maintenance while grasping an object [4, 5] and maintaining a single leg standing position on a rough surface [6, 7]. During these tasks, the attention focus can be directed externally via showing the participant the COP cursor measured by the stabilometer or instructing the participant to keep the object as still as possible. In contrast, the attention focus can be directed internally by focusing the grasping hand or the entire body during posture control. A previous study that examined the effects of attention focus during balance tasks reported the positive effects of external focus [8]. The effects of attention focus during postural control tasks have also been examined in elderly participants [9], in which the same positive motor learning effects are observed. Elderly people often suffer fractures due to falls and require rehabilitation [10]. Therefore, it is expected that external focus can promote the improvement of postural control during rehabilitation for fall prevention.

The effects of internal focus and external focus have also been examined during sports activities that do not require open skill, such as golf putting, dart shooting, and basketball free throws. In golf putting, internal focus directs attention to the arm or the putting motion and external focus directs attention to the golf club or the course of the ball. Several studies have reported more favorable motor learning via external focus than when internal focus or control conditions are used [11, 12]. External focus improves putting accuracy, kinematic parameters [13], and muscle activity as measured by electromyography (EMG) [14], as it smooths the putting motion and decreases muscle activity in the lower extremities. Less muscle activity is required to complete efficient movements. These results indicate that external focus promotes accurate and efficient golf putting. Similar results have been reported regarding the effects of external focus on motor learning during dart shooting and basketball free throws. Internal focus was directed to the participant's wrists and hands, while external focus was directed to the dart trajectory (during dart shooting) or the basket (during basketball free throws). External focus increased movement accuracy, improved kinematic parameters, and decreased muscle activity in both activities [15–17], suggesting that external focus is efficient for motor learning of sports movements that require accuracy and may contribute to the acquisition of more accurate movements. Therefore, verbal instructions regarding external focus may be effective for the rehabilitation of athletes.

1.3 The effects of attention focus on muscle strength and endurance

The effects of attention focus on muscle strength [18], muscular endurance [19], and tasks requiring accuracy have been reported. Several studies have reported short-term gains in muscle strength when external focus is used. External focus increased muscle strength during grip strength [20] and squat and deadlift [21] activities. In addition to muscle strength, changes in muscle activity (measured using EMG) have also been reported [22], suggesting that unnecessary muscle activity during movement is reduced by external focus, promoting more efficient movements. These findings also indicate that the use of external focus results in efficient exercises that encourage selective participation of the muscle groups necessary for the movement. Therefore, muscle strengthening training should be conducted using external focus. However, a previous study reported decreased muscle activity but no improvement in muscle strength when the same muscle force was exerted [23]. No study has reported the positive effects of consistent external focus, and there is no clear difference between internal focus and external focus when examining the long-term effects of training. However, when limited to the lower limb, muscle strength training using external focus has resulted in more favorable outcomes. One study [24] reported the positive effects of internal focus. Therefore, although there is currently no evidence to actively recommend external focus, there is a high possibility that the use of external focus provides more favorable muscle strengthening than internal focus. Patients undergoing rehabilitation due to orthopedic, cardiovascular, or other medical diseases often suffer muscle weakness due to disuse, and require efficient muscle strengthening training. Training using external focus is preferred for muscle strengthening training during rehabilitation.

The positive effects of external focus on muscular endurance have also been reported in several studies. Studies including repetitive exercises using the upper extremities, such as push-ups [20] and bench presses [25], and repetitive exercises using the lower extremities, such as squats and deadlifts [22, 26] have been reported. External focus is used to direct attention to the object during tasks that require the use of heavy objects, such as bench presses and squats. For tasks that do not require the use of an object, such as push-ups, the participants' attention is directed to the external environment, and the participants are instructed to "push on the floor." External focus has been reported to decrease the perception of fatigue and muscle tiredness [27] and it decreases muscle activity when the same muscle force is exerted [22], allowing for more efficient exercise. Increased efficiency prolongs the time to muscle fatigue. The long-term effects of attention focus on improving muscle endurance have not been examined and remain unclear. However, the short-term improvement in muscle endurance when external focus is used allows for more training sessions, resulting in more efficient training for the improvement of muscle strength and endurance. Patients undergoing rehabilitation often have weakened muscular endurance and strength. Therefore, the use of external focus is an efficient method for improving muscle strength and endurance during rehabilitation.

1.4 Dominance of attention focus

The dominance of attention focus has been reported recently as some individuals are internal focus-dominant and others are external focus-dominant. The relationships between abilities and the dominance of attention focus have been examined. Perkins-Ceccato et al. [28] reported that the dominance of attention focus depends on performance during a golf putting task, as a highly-skilled group had a better performance using external focus and a low-skill group had a better performance using internal focus. These results may be due to the fact that the low-skill group must pay attention to each step of the movement to perform it accurately. While beginners need to pay attention to the movement, external focus diverts their attention to the external environment. Participants in the low-skill group may have had insufficient attentional capacity to perform unfamiliar movements when external focus was used, resulting in a worse performance than that of the external focus group. Therefore, internal focus is effective in low-skill groups. Sakurada et al. [29] reported that the dominance of attention focus depends on the motor imagery ability in upper limb tracking tasks. The modality of motor imagery ability includes motor sensory imagery ability and visuomotor imagery ability. Participants with high motor-sensory imagery ability (motor-sensory dominant group) had more favorable motor learning using internal focus while participants with high visual imagery ability (visual dominant group) had more favorable motor learning using external focus. The modality of motor imagery ability and the dominance of attention focus are correlated. Therefore, the effects of internal focus were improved when the polarity of motor sensory dominance was increased. In contrast, the effects of external focus were improved when the polarity of visual dominance was increased. The cortical localization required in motor imagery and attention focus tasks is similar, which may account for the association between the modality of motor imagery ability and the dominance of attention focus. In the previous study, the motor-sensory dominant group had experience in sports that required closed skill, such as swimming and track and field. The visual dominant group had experience in sports that required open skill, such as volleyball and basketball. Therefore, the results of the study may be influenced by the participants' experiences with motor learning and sports training. The visual-dominant group was much larger than the motor-sensory-dominant group [30], suggesting that the observed positive effects of external focus may be due to the difference in group size. Performing tasks with optimal attention strategies leads to better performance, improvement, and promotes motor learning effects. During rehabilitation, therapists are required to tailor interventions to individual patients, and interventions that consider the patient's dominance of attention focus may improve the efficiency of rehabilitation. However, few studies regarding the dominance of attention focus have been reported and the results are inconsistent. Therefore, factors that determine the dominance of attention focus should be identified in future studies, and a scale to assess the dominance of attention focus should be developed.

1.5 Summary

The definitions of internal focus and external focus and the effects of attention focus during various movements based on previous studies that included healthy participants have been described. External focus is thought to be effective to promote the automaticity of movement during rehabilitation. However, the dominance of attention focus requires additional research. The consideration of the optimal attentional focus for patients during rehabilitation interventions will lead to effective and individualized rehabilitation services.

2. Neural basis of internal focus and external focus

Several studies have reported that brain function is related to performance [31–33] and motor learning [33–35]. Similarly, attention focus, which influences performance and motor learning, is expected to be related to brain function. Recently, encephalography (EEG), functional magnetic resonance imaging (fMRI), and functional near-infrared spectroscopy (fNIRS) have been used to examine the neural basis of attention focus. An understanding of the neural basis will not only clarify the existence of attention focus but will also be useful to consider new intervention methods for the modulation of brain activity via neuromodulation and other techniques.

2.1 Neural basis of attention focus

The neural basis of attention focus remains unclear. However, several reports have considered differences in brain functions as related to information processing and cognitive control. Raisbeck et al. [36] used fMRI to examine the effects of attention focus and the differences between internal focus and external focus during knee flexion and extension movements and found that internal focus activates motor-related areas (primary motor cortex and primary somatosensory cortex) and the cerebellar folium vermis. The use of internal focus increases the processing of somatosensory information and the activation of motor-sensory areas. The cerebellar folium vermis is active in internal cognition [37]. The activation of the cerebellar folium vermis may indicate increased cognitive demands. Internal focus increases cognitive demands as it promotes conscious control of the body. In contrast, activation of the anterior part of the lingual gyrus, occipital pole, occipital spindle gyrus, and parahippocampal gyrus was observed when external focus was used. The lingual gyrus and occipital pole are located in the occipital lobe and are involved in the processing of visual information [38]. The occipital spindle gyrus is involved in object recognition. The activation of these three regions indicates an increase in visual information due to the use of external focus. Furthermore, the parahippocampal gyrus is associated with visual memory [39], indicating visually dominant control with external focus. Another study that used EEG reported that external focus activates visual areas [40]. However, additional studies [40, 41] have reported that external focus activates motor-sensory areas, which is inconsistent with the results of the study by Raisbeck et al. [36]. The activation of motor-sensory areas by external focus is caused by the integration of visual and somatosensory information. The increase in visual information due to the use of external focus further increases the somatosensory information, activating the motor-sensory area during the processing of this information. This effect is related to the improvement of performance. Another area associated with this cognitive control is the activity of the frontal region. High theta wave activity in the frontal region of the EEG (FMθ) has been observed during concentration in cognitive tasks [42]. FMθ is also observed when external focus is used [40] and may reflect the effects of attention focus.

The neural basis of attention focus is based on previous studies that have considered the brain regions activated by internal focus and external focus to support function. However, several studies have suggested that the inactivation of brain regions or brain activity similar to that at rest may be efficient. Kuhn et al. [43] used transcranial magnetic stimulation (TMS) to examine the effects of attention focus and the intracortical inhibition of the primary motor cortex and found that external focus improves performance and activates inhibitory circuits in the primary motor cortex. The activity of the intracortical inhibitory circuits indicates the suppression of cortical activity, which may indicate that the suppression of unnecessary brain activity when external focus is used leads to the efficient execution of locally-activated cortical movements. Intracortical inhibition has also been shown to affect motor control, including coordinated movements [44]. Intracortical inhibition may represent the difference in motor control during internal focus and external focus. Therefore, both the activation and inactivation of brain regions may represent the neural basis of attention focus.

2.2 Neural basis of the dominance of attention focus

The neural basis of the dominance of attention focus has also been studied as differences in brain activity due to differences in optimal attention focus existing among individuals. Brain activity in participants using internal focus and those using external focus differed in a study in which participants were divided into internal focus-dominant and external focus-dominant groups based on their performance during an attention-focused task. The neural basis for the dominance of attention focus is related to information processing, cognitive processes, and the neural basis for attention focus. In a study using fNIRS, Sakurada et al. [45] reported that the right dorsolateral prefrontal cortex and somatosensory association cortex were less active in the internal focus-dominant and external focus-dominant groups when performing tasks at optimal attention focus (**Figure 1**). Participants with higher motor skills are able to perform movements with less neural activity than those with lower motor skills [46]. The dorsolateral prefrontal cortex and somatosensory association cortex are responsible for the integration of information and had low activity in this study, suggesting that the optimal attentional strategy enabled movement with less neural activity and less information processing, which indicate efficient brain activity. Furthermore, validation studies regarding event-related potentials using tactile and visual stimuli [47] and fNIRS [48] reported a relationship between the dominance of attention focus and processing of visual and tactile information, supporting the association between information processing and attention focus. In another study [49], EEG was used to examine the neural basis of the dominance of attention focus during a standing, postural control task (**Figure 2**). When internal focus was used, the left parietal lobe

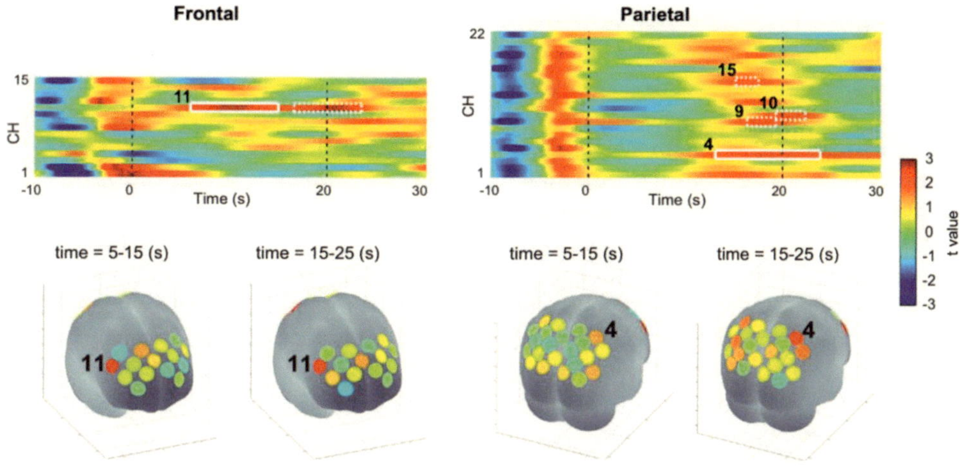

Figure 1.
Differences in brain activity in the optimal attentional strategy [45]. The red area in the parietal lobe, indicated by 4, is the somatosensory association cortex. The red area in the frontal lobe, indicated by 11, is the right dorsolateral prefrontal cortex. These two regions showed inactivity during optimal attentional focus.

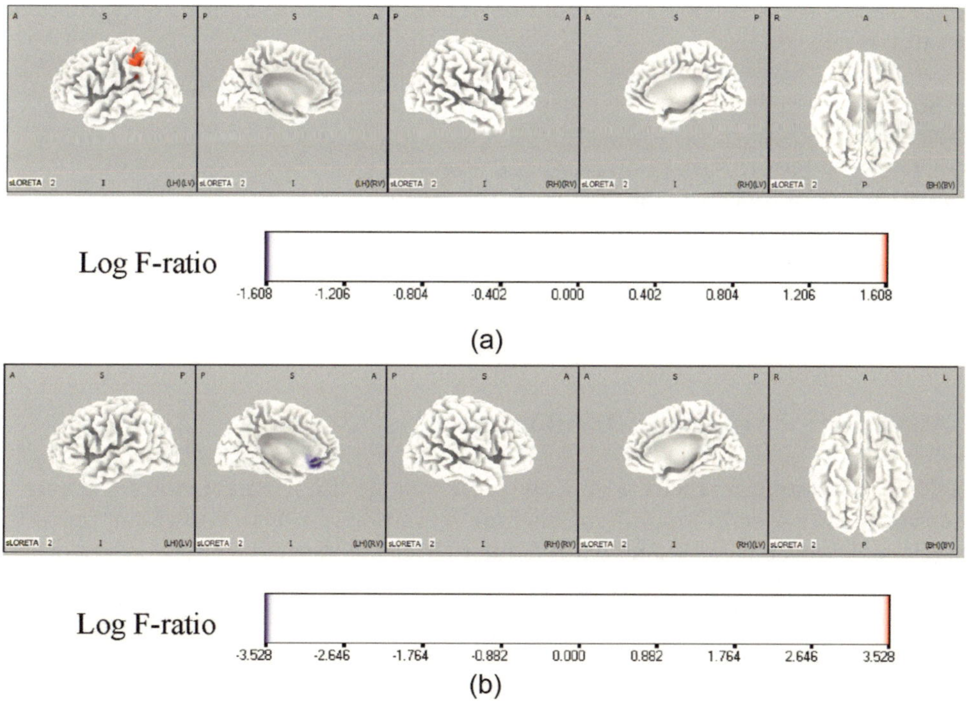

Figure 2.
Differences in EEG activity between the internal focus-dominant group and the external focus-dominant group [49]. The red area is activated in participants in the internal focus-dominant group, while the blue area is activated in participants in the external focus-dominant group. When internal focus is used, the left parietal lobe is hyperactive in the internal focus-dominant group (a). When external focus is used, the left frontal lobe is highly active in the external focus-dominant group (b).

of participants in the internal focus-dominant group had higher theta wave activity. In contrast, the left frontal lobe of participants in the external focus group had higher theta wave activity when external focus was used. High theta wave activity in the parietal lobe has been reported to be associated with the processing of proprioceptive and superficial sensory information [50] and with attentional control [51]. Therefore, the internal focus-dominant group may have increased superficial sensory processing when internal focus is used and may have higher attentional control when directing attention to the inside of the body. In contrast, high theta wave activity in the frontal lobe has been reported to be associated with error detection [52] and cognitive control [53]. Therefore, the external focus-dominant group is more likely to selectively pay attention to the outside of the body when external focus is used and may perform postural control by error detection based on visual information. Studies regarding the neural basis of the dominance of attention focus indicate that sensory processing and cognitive processes are involved.

The results of these studies are contradictory as to whether higher or lower brain activity is more favorable. Some studies have reported that higher brain activity improves information processing [54] and cognitive control [55] by activating more neurons. However, during motor learning [56] and movement mastery [46], lower brain activity has been reported to imply more efficient neural activity. These studies also reported that optimal attentional strategies generated less brain activity and efficient neural activity, while greater neural activity resulted in better performance. Although it is clear that there is a difference in brain activity, further research is needed.

2.3 Summary

The neural bases of attention focus and attention focus dominance involve sensory information processing and cognitive processes. Changes in performance and motor learning due to attention focus occur in the same environment. Therefore, performance and brain activity change based on how information is processed and perceived. The ability to process information and cognitive control may determine the effects of attentional focus.

3. Attention focus during rehabilitation

The use of attention focus to improve performance and promote motor learning does not require specific equipment, making it extremely easy to implement in clinical trials. However, there is a high induction to internal focus during stroke rehabilitation [57], especially with feedback to patients, which is mainly internal focus [58, 59]. Therefore, attention focus may not be considered during rehabilitation. In addition to basic research regarding attention focus, clinical research has shown how rehabilitation can be conducted more effectively via the incorporation of attention focus. In this section, the effects of attention focus on patients with specific diseases are described.

3.1 Attention focus in patients with stroke

The effects of attention focus in patients with stroke have been examined during tasks such as upper limb movement, gait, and postural control. These tasks are related to movements that are impaired by stroke and that impede the return to home and social reintegration. The effects of attention focus have been examined during some accuracy-requiring tasks. More clinical studies have been conducted in patients with stroke with impaired dexterity than in patients with other diseases, and external focus has been reported as effective for patients with stroke. Gomes et al. [60] examined the effects of attention focus during upper limb tasks performed by patients with stroke. The temporal data acquisition instrument (TDAI) [61], an upper limb function test for patients with stroke, was used. The patients' upper limb movements were captured using a camera, and the upper limb movement time, speed, and peak speed were calculated. The results indicate that internal focus and external focus promote motor learning compared to no instructions regarding attention focus in these patients. However, there were no differences in motor learning effects when internal focus or external focus were used. Patient performance is improved when external focus is performed after internal focus as patients with stroke are more likely to exercise conscious control of their movements [62]. Conversely, there was no improvement in performance when internal focus was used after external focus. This indicates that external focus suppresses conscious control of movement and improves performance. A negative correlation between conscious control and motor function has been reported in patients with stroke, and patient function improves when the patients depart from conscious control. As internal focus promotes the conscious control of movements [63, 64], it may be effective during early rehabilitation in patients with stroke who tend to exercise conscious control. Therefore, no differences in motor learning were found when internal focus or external focus were used. However, no reports regarding the relationship between the stage and severity of stroke and the dominance of attention focus have been reported. As the benefits of verbally instructing patients with stroke to pay attention during upper limb movements are clear, these patients should be instructed to pay attention to their upper limbs and the environment, instead of simply performing repetitive movements.

Kim et al. [65] reported that external focus increased step and stride lengths, walking speed, and load on the paralyzed leg when employed during walking in stroke patients. In this study, the subjects' attention was directed to their lower limbs in the internal focus condition and to a line drawn on the floor in the external focus condition. The results indicate that external focus not only improves gait parameters such as step length, but also promote loading of the paralyzed lower extremity. This may be due to the fact that external focus promotes automatic gait control, resulting in a gait pattern similar to normal gait, which in turn promotes loading of the paralyzed lower limb. This is also important for the acquisition of symmetrical and stable gait [66], and the gait speed may have been improved by adopting a gait pattern similar to normal gait. In the rehabilitation of stroke patients, walking ability is an important factor that determines the outcome [67] and the patient's level of living [68]. In addition, it has been reported that gait training for chronic stroke patients does not produce sufficient evidence for functional recovery [69], and efficient improvement of walking ability during the recovery phase is required. Furthermore, it is necessary to acquire automaticity of movements by various tasks for walking in stroke patients [68], and we believe that automating movements with external focus based on the restricted action hypothesis (CAH) is effective. Based on the above, we recommend an efficient intervention with external focus to improve walking ability in stroke patients.

Aloraini et al. [70] compared kinematic data obtained via motion capture and physiological data obtained via EMG during a step postural control task performed by patients with stroke using attention focus. The step task was performed under various step distance and step landing area conditions. When external focus was used, the body movement time, higher peak velocity, and time to peak velocity were shorter and the sway in the final position was smaller. The timing of muscle contraction was faster and the muscle contractions were smaller when external focus was used. Smaller muscle contractions indicate more efficient movements. These results indicate that external focus is effective for postural control in patients with stroke.

The effects of attention focus on motor learning during postural control tasks have also been reported. Kal et al. [71] examined the long-term effects of attention focus during postural control tasks in patients with stroke and found that although external focus improves performance in the short term, there were no significant differences between the long-term effects of internal focus and external focus. However, external focus was effective for patients with stroke who had improved balance, good sensory function, and a small attention capacity, indicating that the interventions should be tailored to individuals based on their optimal attention focus. These results agree with those of Perkins-Ceccato [28], who reported that external focus is effective in patients with high ability, and in an additional study [49] that reported that an internal focus-dominant group has high attentional control ability based on EEG activity. However, few studies have examined the long-term effects of attention focus, and sufficient evidence has not been obtained. More research is necessary. In addition, the symptoms of stroke vary according to the location of the lesion, and the effects and dominance of attention focus may differ based on the stroke symptoms. Therefore, more studies regarding the effects of attention focus in patients with different stroke symptoms are needed. Patients with stroke often suffer from impaired balance due to trunk dysfunction [72], and rehabilitation often includes interventions to improve balance ability [73]. Recently, virtual reality (VR) training [74–76] and electrical stimulation [77] have been investigated as new intervention methods for postural control in patients with stroke. Although these new intervention methods have been reported as effective, they require specific equipment and are difficult to implement in some situations. In comparison, attention focus can improve the postural control using only verbal instruction from therapists and requires no equipment or cost. Therefore, attention focus is clinically useful, and interventions should be conducted to promote performance and motor learning while seeking the optimal attention focus for postural control in patients with stroke.

The effects of attention focus on patients with stroke are not consistent. However, no studies have reported more favorable results without the use of attention focus compared to with the use of attention focus. Therefore, not considering the patient's attention focus may impede performance improvement. The use of the patient's optimal attention focus may lead to improved performance during the rehabilitation of patients with stroke.

3.2 Attention focus in patients with Parkinson's disease

The effects of attention focus in patients with Parkinson's disease have been examined during postural control and gait tasks. The main symptoms of Parkinson's disease are tremors, rigidity, immobility, and impaired postural reflexes [78]. Impaired postural reflexes lead to decreased gait ability, resulting in decreased activities of daily living (ADL) [79]. Therefore, effective treatment methods for postural control and gait are essential for patients with Parkinson's disease. Paradoxical gait [80] triggered by auditory or visual information is a well-known characteristic of Parkinson's disease. Therefore, the performance of patients with Parkinson's disease can be improved via exercises based on information from the environment. The use of external focus has positive effects in patients with Parkinson's disease. Wulf et al. [81] studied the effects of attention focus during a standing posture control task on an unstable surface performed by patients with Parkinson's disease and found that the use of external focus reduced postural sway compared to the control condition and the use of internal focus. Patients with Parkinson's disease may have impaired endogenous regulation derived from the basal ganglia [82], resulting in poor performance during the use of internal focus. Therefore, the use of external focus is recommended for postural control training in patients with Parkinson's disease during rehabilitation.

Beck et al. [83] also examined the effects of attention focus on gait during a dual-task in patients with Parkinson's disease. The use of external focus decreased the step time, while the use of internal focus decreased the step length and gait speed, suggesting that external focus promotes automaticity during dual-task gait and that internal focus impairs the dual-task gait. The unified Parkinson's disease rating scale motor section (UPDRS subsection III) was lower when external focus was used, indicating that external focus improves motor dysfunction caused by Parkinson's disease. However, another study [84] reported increase in walking speed and stride length when internal focus was used, and that these improvements occurred without compromising the performance of the dual-task. The positive effects of internal focus are related to the pathogenesis of Parkinson's disease. Parkinson's disease causes a loss of automaticity in learned movements due to damage to the basal ganglia. Therefore, the use of external focus is less effective as it attempts to use reduced automaticity to perform movements, and conscious control (the use of internal focus) may be effective as a compensation for the loss of automaticity. In summary, both internal focus and external focus have been reported to be effective to improve gait in patients with Parkinson's disease, even when the pathophysiology of Parkinson's disease is considered. However, it is interesting to note that performance is changed by attention focus. It is necessary to clarify whether attention focus should be used to improve lost abilities or to promote the compensatory use of remaining abilities in patients with Parkinson's disease.

The effects of attention focus on patients with Parkinson's disease remain unclear. The relationship between attention focus and brain function requires further research. The effects of attention focus on patients with Parkinson's disease may be revealed via future basic research as Parkinson's disease is a neurodegenerative disease.

3.3 Attention focus in patients with orthopedic diseases

The effects of attention focus on patients with orthopedic diseases have been examined mainly in patients with anterior cruciate ligament (ACL) injuries [85]. ACL injuries are classified into contact and non-contact types. The non-contact type is caused by the force exerted on the knee joint during movements such as landing a jump or stepping [86–89] and accounts for 70–75% of ACL injuries [90]. In patients with non-contact ACL injuries, safe landing is effective in preventing re-tears. The appropriate motor acquisition through motor learning is necessary after a non-contact ACL injury, and improving the efficiency of motor learning using attention focus is of great significance in the rehabilitation of patients with ACL injuries. Gokeler et al. [91] investigated the effects of attention focus on kinematic indices for single-leg jumping movements in patients after ACL reconstruction (ACLR) and found that safe landing movements (including the knee flexion angle at contact; peak knee flexion angle; total range of motion of the hip, knee, and ankle joints in the sagittal plane;

and time to peak knee flexion angle) were significantly higher when external focus was used. However, this study examined temporary performance, and the motor learning effects are not clear. Appropriate movements are necessary for motor learning, and these movements are acquired through repetition. Therefore, movement training with the use of external focus is recommended during the rehabilitation of patients after ACLR.

Attention focus can also be used for ACL injury prevention [92, 93]. ACL injury prevention training reduces the risk of ACL injury [94] and improves the training of soccer players. The effects of attention focus on ACL injury prevention can be inferred from the kinematic effects of squatting in healthy participants. Benjaminse et al. [95] recommended interventions using external focus during single-leg squat and lunge movements. External focus has been shown to result in less knee joint eversion that can lead to ACL injuries. The use of repetitive movements that do not cause knee joint eversion may contribute to ACL injury prevention.

The effects of external focus are clearer in patients with musculoskeletal diseases than in patients with neurological diseases [96]. The contradictory findings regarding the use of attention focus in patients with neurological diseases may be related to brain function in attention focus. The lack of direct brain damage in patients with orthopedic injuries may account for similar effects of attention focus in these patients and in healthy participants. Although the effects of attention focus should be carefully examined and implemented in clinical practice, interventions using external focus are recommended, especially for patients with musculoskeletal disorders.

3.4 Attention focus in patients with developmental disabilities

The effects of attention focus in patients with developmental disabilities have been examined mainly in patients with developmental coordination disorder (DCD). DCD cannot be explained by general intellectual disabilities or specific congenital or acquired neurological disorders alone [97, 98]. Although several studies have shown the effectiveness of exercise therapy for patients with DCD [99–102], there are reports of a lack of automaticity in movement [103], and additional intervention methods are needed. Jarus et al. [104] examined the effects of attention focus on motor learning effects in patients with DCD and in normally-developing children and found that normally-developing children had good retention of learning when external focus was used, though no significant difference was found between the use of internal focus and external focus in patients with DCD. These findings may be due to the fact that patients with DCD are unable to follow instructions accurately and have a lack of concentration and interest and do not indicate that attention focus is ineffective for patients with DCD. Internal focus and external focus may not be used appropriately in these patients as it is difficult for them to pay attention to a forced motor learning task, and patients with DCD are more likely to experience decreased concentration and effort due to repeated failures [105]. Therefore, experimental tasks such as repetitive movements may not be performed appropriately, and the effects of attention focus are difficult to study. Additional studies [106, 107] have reported that the use of external focus is as effective in patients with DCD as in normally-developing children. However, the data of patients DCD and normally-developing children were combined in these studies and were not verified using the data of patients with DCD alone. Therefore, the effects of attention focus on patients with DCD remain unclear and should be reexamined in future studies. The effects of attention focus on motor learning that can improve the motor skills of patients with DCD must also be investigated.

3.5 Summary

The effects of attention focus on patients with various disease have been studied. During rehabilitation, it is necessary to improve the movement ability and to promote motor learning. The clinical usefulness of attention focus to change those abilities is apparent. However, the study findings were inconsistent and should be interpreted with care. Further research is needed to clarify whether attention focus is disease-dependent or homeostatic.

4. Conclusion

In this chapter, the effects of internal focus and external focus on brain activity, performance, and motor learning are summarized. The effects of attention focus are unclear. However, the use of attention focus has the potential to improve patient performance during rehabilitation without the need for special equipment. Based on conflicting findings, both internal focus and external focus should be implemented during rehabilitation, and the most optimal attention focus for individual patients should be considered. The inclusion of attention focus during rehabilitation will make physical therapists' interventions more effective.

Acknowledgements

We would like to thank Editage (www.editage.com) for English language editing. This work was supported by the Yuumi Memorial Foundation for Home Health Care and JSPS KAKENHI Grant Number JP20K11173.

Conflict of interest

The authors declare no conflicts of interest.

Appendices and nomenclature

EMG	electromyography
EEG	electroencephalography
fMRI	functional magnetic resonance imaging
CAH	constrained action hypothesis
COP	center of pressure
fNIRS	functional near-infrared spectroscopy
TMS	transcranial magnetic stimulation
TDAI	temporal data acquisition instrument
VR	virtual reality
ADL	activity of daily living
UPDRS	unified Parkinson's disease rating scale
ACL	anterior cruciate ligament
ACLR	anterior cruciate ligament reconstruction
DCD	developmental coordination disorder

Author details

Shun Sawai[1,2], Shoya Fujikawa[3], Ryosuke Yamamoto[4] and Hideki Nakano[1*]

1 Neurorehabilitation Laboratory, Graduate School of Health Sciences, Kyoto Tachibana University, Kyoto, Japan

2 Department of Rehabilitation, Kyoto Kuno Hospital, Kyoto, Japan

3 Neurorehabilitation Laboratory, Faculty of Health Sciences, Department of Physical Therapy, Kyoto Tachibana University, Kyoto, Japan

4 Department of Rehabilitation, Tesseikai Neurosurgical Hospital, Osaka, Japan

*Address all correspondence to: nakano-h@tachibana-u.ac.jp

IntechOpen

© 2022 The Author(s). Licensee IntechOpen. This chapter is distributed under the terms of the Creative Commons Attribution License (http://creativecommons.org/licenses/by/3.0), which permits unrestricted use, distribution, and reproduction in any medium, provided the original work is properly cited.

References

[1] Wulf G, Höß M, Prinz W. Instructions for motor learning: Differential effects of internal versus external focus of attention. Journal of Motor Behavior. 1998;**30**:169-179. DOI: 10.1080/00222899809601334

[2] Wulf G, McNevin N, Shea CH. The automaticity of complex motor skill learning as a function of attentional focus. The Quarterly Journal of Experimental Psychology Section A. 2001;**54**:1143-1154. DOI: 10.1080/713756012

[3] Wulf G, Töllner T, Shea CH. Attentional focus effects as a function of task difficulty. Research Quarterly for Exercise and Sport. 2007;**78**:257-264. DOI: 10.1080/02701367.2007.10599423

[4] Cluff T, Gharib T, Balasubramaniam R. Attentional influences on the performance of secondary physical tasks during posture control. Experimental Brain Research. 2010;**203**:647-658. DOI: 10.1007/s00221-010-2274-7

[5] Wulf G, Weigelt M, Poulter D, McNevin N. Attentional focus on suprapostural tasks affects balance learning. The Quarterly Journal of Experimental Psychology Section A. 2003;**56**:1191-1211. DOI: 10.1080/02724980343000062

[6] Wulf G. Attentional focus effects in balance acrobats. Research Quarterly for Exercise and Sport. 2008;**79**:319-325. DOI: 10.1080/02701367.2008.10599495

[7] Wulf G, Mercer J, McNevin N, Guadagnoli MA. Reciprocal influences of attentional focus on postural and suprapostural task performance. Journal of Motor Behavior. 2004;**36**:189-199. DOI: 10.3200/JMBR.36.2.189-199

[8] Aloraini SM, Gelley G, Glazebrook C, Sibley KM, Singer J, Passmore S. Motor behavior concepts in the study of balance: A scoping review. Journal of Motor Behavior. 2020;**52**:97-121. DOI: 10.1080/00222895.2019.1582472

[9] Chiviacowsky S, Wulf G, Wally R. An external focus of attention enhances balance learning in older adults. Gait & Posture. 2010;**32**:572-575. DOI: 10.1016/j.gaitpost.2010.08.004

[10] Kalache A, Fu D, Yoshida S, Al-Faisal W, Beattie L, Chodzko-Zajko W, Fu H, James K, Kalula S, Krishnaswamy B, Kronfol N, Marin P, Pike I, Rose D, Scott V, Stevens J, Todd C, Usha G, Ageing DO, Course L. World Health Organisation Global Report on Falls Prevention in Older Age. Available from: http://www.who.int/ageing/publications/Falls_prevention7March.pdf [Accessed: April 4, 2022]

[11] Wulf G, Su J. An external focus of attention enhances golf shot accuracy in beginners and experts. Research Quarterly for Exercise and Sport. 2007;**78**:384-389. DOI: 10.1080/02701367.2007.10599436

[12] Shafizadeh M, McMorris T, Sproule J. Effect of different external attention of focus instruction on learning of golf putting skill. Perceptual and Motor Skills. 2011;**113**:662-670. DOI: 10.2466/05.23.25.PMS.113.5.662-670

[13] Munzert J, Maurer H, Reiser M. Verbal-motor attention-focusing instructions influence kinematics and performance on a golf-putting task. Journal of Motor Behavior. 2014;**46**:309-318. DOI: 10.1080/00222895.2014.912197

[14] Pelleck V, Passmore SR. Location versus task relevance: The impact of differing internal focus of attention instructions on motor performance. Acta Psychologica. 2017;**176**:23-31. DOI: 10.1016/j.actpsy.2017.03.007

[15] Lohse KR, Sherwood DE, Healy AF. How changing the focus of attention affects performance, kinematics, and electromyography in dart throwing. Human Movement Science. 2010;**29**:542-555. DOI: 10.1016/j.humov.2010.05.001

[16] Hitchcock DR, Sherwood DE. Effects of changing the focus of attention on accuracy, acceleration, and electromyography in dart throwing. International Journal of Exercise Science. 2018;**11**:1120-1135

[17] Zachry T, Wulf G, Mercer J, Bezodis N. Increased movement accuracy and reduced EMG activity as the result of adopting an external focus of attention. Brain Research Bulletin. 2005;**67**:304-309. DOI: 10.1016/j.brainresbull.2005.06.035

[18] Grgic J, Mikulic I, Mikulic P. Acute and long-term effects of attentional focus strategies on muscular strength: A Meta-analysis. Sports (Basel). 2021;**9**:153. DOI: 10.3390/sports9110153

[19] Grgic J, Mikulic P. Effects of attentional focus on muscular endurance: A Meta-analysis. International Journal of Environmental Research and Public Health. 2021;**19**:89. DOI: 10.3390/ijerph19010089

[20] Bredin SS, Dickson DB, Warburton DE. Effects of varying attentional focus on health-related physical fitness performance. Applied Physiology, Nutrition, and Metabolism. 2013;**38**:161-168. DOI: 10.1139/apnm-2012-0182

[21] Nadzalan AM, Lee JLF, Azzfar MS, Muhammad NS, Shukri EWMC, Mohamad NI. The effects of resistance training with different focus attention on muscular strength: Application to teaching methods in physical conditioning class. In: J Phys.: Conf. Ser.; 25-27 November 2019. Bandung: JICETS; 2019. pp. 16-19

[22] Nadzalan A, Low J, Mohamad NI, Mohamad AM, Abd MN, Mohamad CEW. The effects of focus attention instructions on the movement kinetics, muscle activation and performance during resistance exercise. Journal of Physics: Conference Series. 2020;**1529**:022008. DOI: 10.1088/1742-6596/1529/2/022008

[23] Marchant DC, Greig M. Attentional focusing instructions influence quadriceps activity characteristics but not force production during isokinetic knee extensions. Human Movement Science. 2017;**52**:67-73. DOI: 10.1016/j.humov.2017.01.007

[24] Schoenfeld BJ, Vigotsky A, Contreras B, Golden S, Alto A, Larson R, et al. Differential effects of attentional focus strategies during long-term resistance training. European Journal of Sport Science. 2018;**18**:705-712. DOI: 10.1080/17461391.2018.1447020

[25] Collum C, Snarr R, Siekirk N, Wilson S. Effects of attentional focus on repetitions-to-failure & motor unit excitation during submaximal bench press performance. International Journal of Strength and Conditioning. 2021;**1**:1-12. DOI: 10.47206/ijsc.v1i1.35

[26] Nadzalan A, Low J, Mohamad NI. The effects of focus attention instructions on strength training performances. International Journal of Humanities and Management

Sciences. 2015;**3**:418-423. DOI: 10.1088/1742-6596/1529/2/022008

[27] Lohse KR, Sherwood DE. Defining the focus of attention: Effects of attention on perceived exertion and fatigue. Frontiers in Psychology. 2011;**2**:332. DOI: 10.3389/fpsyg.2011.00332

[28] Perkins-Ceccato N, Passmore SR, Lee TD. Effects of focus of attention depend on golfers' skill. Journal of Sports Sciences. 2003;**21**:593-600. DOI: 10.1080/0264041031000101980

[29] Sakurada T, Hirai M, Watanabe E. Optimization of a motor learning attention-directing strategy based on an individual's motor imagery ability. Experimental Brain Research. 2016;**234**:301-311. DOI: 10.1007/s00221-015-4464-9

[30] Malouin F, Richards CL, Jackson PL, Lafleur MF, Durand A, Doyon J. The Kinesthetic and visual imagery questionnaire (KVIQ) for assessing motor imagery in persons with physical disabilities: A reliability and construct validity study. Journal of Neurologic Physical Therapy. 2007;**31**:20-29. DOI: 10.1097/01.npt.0000260567.24122.64

[31] Perrey S, Besson P. Studying brain activity in sports performance: Contributions and issues. Progress in Brain Research. 2018;**240**:247-267. DOI: 10.1016/bs.pbr.2018.07.004

[32] Picazio S, Koch G. Is motor inhibition mediated by cerebello-cortical interactions? Cerebellum. 2015;**14**:47-49. DOI: 10.1007/s12311-014-0609-9

[33] Moore D, Jung M, Hillman CH, Kang M, Loprinzi PD. Interrelationships between exercise, functional connectivity, and cognition among healthy adults: A systematic review. Psychophysiology. 2022;**59**:e14014. DOI: 10.1111/psyp.14014

[34] Halsband U, Lange RK. Motor learning in man: A review of functional and clinical studies. Journal of Physiology, Paris. 2006;**99**:414-424. DOI: 10.1016/j.jphysparis.2006.03.007

[35] Seidler RD, Noll DC. Neuroanatomical correlates of motor acquisition and motor transfer. Journal of Neurophysiology. 2008;**99**:1836-1845. DOI: 10.1152/jn.01187.2007

[36] Raisbeck LD, Diekfuss JA, Grooms DR, Schmitz R. The effects of attentional focus on brain function during a gross motor task. Journal of Sport Rehabilitation. 2019;**29**:441-447. DOI: 10.1123/jsr.2018-0026

[37] Allen G, Buxton RB, Wong EC, Courchesne E. Attentional activation of the cerebellum independent of motor involvement. Science. 1997;**275**:1940-1943. DOI: 10.1126/science.275.5308.1940

[38] Grill-Spector K, Kushnir T, Hendler T, Edelman S, Itzchak Y, Malach R. A sequence of object-processing stages revealed by fMRI in the human occipital lobe. Human Brain Mapping. 1998;**6**:316-328. DOI: 10.1002/(SICI)1097-0193(1998)6:4<316::AID-HBM9>3.0.CO;2-6

[39] Takahashi E, Ohki K, Miyashita Y. The role of the parahippocampal gyrus in source memory for external and internal events. Neuroreport. 2002;**13**:1951-1956. DOI: 10.1097/00001756-200210280-00024

[40] Sherman DA, Lehmann T, Baumeister J, Gokeler A, Donovan L, Norte GE. External focus of attention influences cortical activity associated

with single limb balance performance. Physical Therapy. 2021;**101**:pzab223. DOI: 10.1093/ptj/pzab223

[41] Zentgraf K, Lorey B, Bischoff M, Zimmermann K, Stark R, Munzert J. Neural correlates of attentional focusing during finger movements: A fMRI study. Journal of Motor Behavior. 2009;**41**:535-541. DOI: 10.3200/35-08-091

[42] Eschmann KCJ, Bader R, Mecklinger A. Topographical differences of frontal-midline theta activity reflect functional differences in cognitive control abilities. Brain and Cognition. 2018;**123**:57-64. DOI: 10.1016/j.bandc.2018.02.002

[43] Kuhn YA, Keller M, Ruffieux J, Taube W. Intracortical inhibition within the primary motor cortex can Be modulated by changing the focus of attention. Journal of Visualized Experiments. 2017;**127**:55771. DOI: 10.3791/55771

[44] Fujiyama H, Hinder MR, Schmidt MW, Garry MI, Summers JJ. Age-related differences in corticospinal excitability and inhibition during coordination of upper and lower limbs. Neurobiology of Aging. 2012;**33**:1484.e1-1484.e14. DOI: 10.1016/j.neurobiolaging.2011.12.019

[45] Sakurada T, Hirai M, Watanabe E. Individual optimal attentional strategy during implicit motor learning boosts frontoparietal neural processing efficiency: A functional near-infrared spectroscopy study. Brain and Behavior: A Cognitive Neuroscience Perspective. 2019;**9**:e01183. DOI: 10.1002/brb3.1183

[46] Naito E, Hirose S. Efficient foot motor control by Neymar's brain. Frontiers in Human Neuroscience. 2014;**8**:594. DOI: 10.3389/fnhum.2014.00594

[47] Sakurada T, Yoshida M, Nagai K. Individual optimal attentional strategy in motor learning tasks characterized by steady-state somatosensory and visual evoked potentials. Frontiers in Human Neuroscience. 2022;**15**:784292. DOI: 10.3389/fnhum.2021.784292

[48] Sakurada T, Goto A, Tetsuka M, Nakajima T, Morita M, Yamamoto SI, et al. Prefrontal activity predicts individual differences in optimal attentional strategy for preventing motor performance decline: A functional near-infrared spectroscopy study. Neurophotonics. 2019;**6**:025012. DOI: 10.1117/1.NPh.6.2.025012

[49] Sawai S, Fujikawa S, Murata S, Abiko T, Nakano H. Dominance of attention focus and its electroencephalogram activity in standing postural control in healthy young adults. Brain Sciences. 2022;**12**:538. DOI: 10.3390/brainsci12050538

[50] Reichenbach A, Thielscher A, Peer A, Bülthoff HH, Bresciani JP. A key region in the human parietal cortex for processing proprioceptive hand feedback during reaching movements. NeuroImage. 2014;**84**:615-625. DOI: 10.1016/j.neuroimage.2013.09.024

[51] Huizeling E, Wang H, Holland C, Kessler K. Changes in theta and alpha oscillatory signatures of attentional control in older and middle age. The European Journal of Neuroscience. 2021;**54**:4314-4337. DOI: 10.1111/ejn.15259

[52] Solis-Escalante T, van der Cruijsen J, de Kam D, van Kordelaar J, Weerdesteyn V, Schouten AC. Cortical dynamics during preparation and execution of reactive balance responses with distinct postural demands.

NeuroImage. 2019;**188**:557-571. DOI: 10.1016/j.neuroimage.2018.12.045

[53] Cavanagh JF, Frank MJ. Frontal theta as a mechanism for cognitive control. Trends in Cognitive Sciences. 2014;**18**:414-421. DOI: 10.1016/j.tics.2014.04.012

[54] Vanni S, Sharifian F, Heikkinen H, Vigário R. Modeling fMRI signals can provide insights into neural processing in the cerebral cortex. Journal of Neurophysiology. 2015;**114**:768-780. DOI: 10.1152/jn.00332.2014

[55] Gratton G, Cooper P, Fabiani M, Carter CS, Karayanidis F. Dynamics of cognitive control: Theoretical bases, paradigms, and a view for the future. Psychophysiology. 2018;**55**:e13016. DOI: 10.1111/psyp.13016

[56] Goto K, Hoshi Y, Sata M, Kawahara M, Takahashi M, Murohashi H. Role of the prefrontal cortex in the cognitive control of reaching movements: Near-infrared spectroscopy study. Journal of Biomedical Optics. 2011;**16**:127003. DOI: 10.1117/1.3658757

[57] Johnson L, Burridge JH, Demain SH. Internal and external focus of attention during gait re-education: An observational study of physical therapist practice in stroke rehabilitation. Physical Therapy. 2013;**93**:957-966. DOI: 10.2522/ptj.20120300

[58] Kal E, van den Brink H, Houdijk H, van der Kamp J, Goossens PH, van Bennekom C, et al. How physical therapists instruct patients with stroke: An observational study on attentional focus during gait rehabilitation after stroke. Disability and Rehabilitation. 2018;**40**:1154-1165. DOI: 10.1080/09638288.2017.1290697

[59] Durham K, Van Vliet PM, Badger F, Sackley C. Use of information feedback and attentional focus of feedback in treating the person with a hemiplegic arm. Physiotherapy Research International. 2009;**14**:77-90. DOI: 10.1002/pri.431

[60] Gomes CLA, Cacho RO, Nobrega VTB, Galvão F, de Araújo DS, Medeiros ALS, et al. Effects of attentional focus on upper extremity motor performance in post stroke patients: A randomized pilot study. Medicine (Baltimore). 2021;**100**:e24656. DOI: 10.1097/MD.0000000000024656

[61] Gomes CLA, Cacho RO, Nobrega VTB, de A Confessor EM, de, EEM F, JLF N, et al. Low-cost equipment for the evaluation of reach and grasp in post-stroke individuals: A pilot study. Biomedical Engineering Online. 2020;**19**:14. DOI: 10.1186/s12938-020-0758-7

[62] Orrell AJ, Masters RS, Eves FF. Reinvestment and movement disruption following stroke. Neurorehabilitation and Neural Repair. 2009;**23**:177-183. DOI: 10.1177/1545968308317752

[63] Mak TCT, Wong TWL. Do attentional focus instructions affect real-time reinvestment during level-ground walking in older adults? Cognitive Processing. 2022;**23**:121-128. DOI: 10.1007/s10339-021-01044-3

[64] Law JCL, Wong TWL. Internal focus instruction increases psychological stress with conscious motor processing and deteriorates motor performance in dart throwing. Cognitive Processing. 2021;**22**:57-64. DOI: 10.1007/s10339-020-00991-7

[65] Kim SA, Ryu YU, Shin HK. The effects of different attentional focus on poststroke gait. Journal of Exercise

Rehabilitation. 2019;**15**:592-596. DOI: 10.12965/jer.1938360.180

[66] Zhang W, Smuck M, Legault C, Ith MA, Muaremi A, Aminian K. Gait symmetry assessment with a Low Back 3D accelerometer in post-stroke patients. Sensors (Basel). 2018;**18**:3322. DOI: 10.3390/s18103322

[67] Han P, Zhang W, Kang L, Ma Y, Fu L, Jia L, et al. Clinical evidence of exercise benefits for stroke. Advances in Experimental Medicine and Biology. 2017;**1000**:131-151. DOI: 10.1007/978-981-10-4304-8_9

[68] Beyaert C, Vasa R, Frykberg GE. Gait post-stroke: Pathophysiology and rehabilitation strategies. Neurophysiologie Clinique. 2015;**45**:335-355. DOI: 10.1016/j.neucli.2015.09.005

[69] States RA, Salem Y, Pappas E. Overground gait training for individuals with chronic stroke: A Cochrane systematic review. Journal of Neurologic Physical Therapy. 2009;**33**:179-186. DOI: 10.1097/NPT.0b013e3181c29a8c

[70] Aloraini SM, Glazebrook CM, Pooyania S, Sibley KM, Singer J, Passmore S. An external focus of attention compared to an internal focus of attention improves anticipatory postural adjustments among people post-stroke. Gait & Posture. 2020;**82**:100-105. DOI: 10.1016/j.gaitpost.2020.08.133

[71] Kal E, Houdijk H, van der Kamp J, Verhoef M, Prosée R, Groet E, et al. Are the effects of internal focus instructions different from external focus instructions given during balance training in stroke patients? A double-blind randomized controlled trial. Clinical Rehabilitation. 2019;**33**:207-221. DOI: 10.1177/0269215518795243

[72] Van Criekinge T, Truijen S, Schröder J, Maebe Z, Blanckaert K, van der Waal C, et al. The effectiveness of trunk training on trunk control, sitting and standing balance and mobility post-stroke: A systematic review and meta-analysis. Clinical Rehabilitation. 2019;**33**:992-1002. DOI: 10.1177/0269215519830159

[73] Arienti C, Lazzarini SG, Pollock A, Negrini S. Rehabilitation interventions for improving balance following stroke: An overview of systematic reviews. PLoS One. 2019;**14**:e0219781. DOI: 10.1371/journal.pone.0219781

[74] Chen L, Lo WL, Mao YR, Ding MH, Lin Q, Li H, et al. Effect of virtual reality on postural and balance control in patients with stroke: A systematic literature review. BioMed Research International. 2016;**2016**:7309272. DOI: 10.1155/2016/7309272

[75] Mohammadi R, Semnani AV, Mirmohammadkhani M, Grampurohit N. Effects of virtual reality compared to conventional therapy on balance Poststroke: A systematic review and Meta-analysis. Journal of Stroke and Cerebrovascular Diseases. 2019;**28**:1787-1798. DOI: 10.1016/j.jstrokecerebrovasdis.2019.03.054

[76] Laver KE, Lange B, George S, Deutsch JE, Saposnik G, Crotty M. Virtual reality for stroke rehabilitation. Cochrane Database of Systematic Reviews. 2017;**11**:CD008349. DOI: 10.1002/14651858.CD008349.pub4

[77] Lin S, Sun Q, Wang H, Xie G. Influence of transcutaneous electrical nerve stimulation on spasticity, balance, and walking speed in stroke patients: A systematic review and meta-analysis. Journal of Rehabilitation Medicine. 2018;**50**:3-7. DOI: 10.2340/16501977-2266

[78] Jankovic J. Parkinson's disease: Clinical features and diagnosis. Journal of Neurology, Neurosurgery, and Psychiatry. 2008;**79**:368-376. DOI: 10.1136/jnnp.2007.131045

[79] Tan D, Danoudis M, McGinley J, Morris ME. Relationships between motor aspects of gait impairments and activity limitations in people with Parkinson's disease: A systematic review. Parkinsonism & Related Disorders. 2012;**18**:117-124. DOI: 10.1016/j.parkreldis.2011.07.014

[80] Moreau C, Cantiniaux S, Delval A, Defebvre L, Azulay JP. Les troubles de la marche dans la maladie de Parkinson: problématique clinique et physiopathologique [Gait disorders in Parkinson's disease: and pathophysiological approaches]. Revue Neurologique (Paris). 2010;**166**:158-167. DOI: 10.1016/j.neurol.2009.05.010

[81] Wulf G, Landers M, Lewthwaite R, Töllner T. External focus instructions reduce postural instability in individuals with Parkinson disease. Physical Therapy. 2009;**89**:162-168. DOI: 10.2522/ptj.20080045

[82] Wu T, Hallett M. A functional MRI study of automatic movements in patients with Parkinson's disease. Brain. 2005;**128**:2250-2259. DOI: 10.1093/brain/awh569

[83] Beck EN, Intzandt BN, Almeida QJ. Can dual task walking improve in Parkinson's disease after external focus of attention exercise? A single blind randomized controlled trial. Neurorehabilitation and Neural Repair. 2018;**32**:18-33. DOI: 10.1177/1545968317746782

[84] Beck EN, Wang MTY, Intzandt BN, Almeida QJ, Ehgoetz Martens KA. Sensory focused exercise improves anxiety in Parkinson's disease: A randomized controlled trial. PLoS One. 2020;**15**:e0230803. DOI: 10.1371/journal.pone.0230803

[85] Singh H, Gokeler A, Benjaminse A. Effective attentional focus strategies after anterior cruciate ligament reconstruction: A commentary. International Journal of Sports Physical Therapy. 2021;**16**:1575-1585. DOI: 10.26603/001c.29848

[86] Boden BP, Sheehan FT. Mechanism of non-contact ACL injury: OREF clinical research award 2021. Journal of Orthopaedic Research. 2022;**40**:531-540. DOI: 10.1002/jor.25257

[87] Shimokochi Y, Shultz SJ. Mechanisms of noncontact anterior cruciate ligament injury. Journal of Athletic Training. 2008;**43**:396-408. DOI: 10.4085/1062-6050-43.4.396

[88] Boden BP, Sheehan FT, Torg JS, Hewett TE. Noncontact anterior cruciate ligament injuries: Mechanisms and risk factors. The Journal of the American Academy of Orthopaedic Surgeons. 2010;**18**:520-527. DOI: 10.5435/00124635-201009000-00003

[89] Dauty M, Crenn V, Louguet B, Grondin J, Menu P, Fouasson-Chailloux A. Anatomical and neuromuscular factors associated to non-contact anterior cruciate ligament injury. Journal of Clinical Medicine. 2022;**11**:1402. DOI: 10.3390/jcm11051402

[90] Buckthorpe M. Recommendations for movement Re-training after ACL reconstruction. Sports Medicine. 2021;**51**:1601-1618. DOI: 10.1007/s40279-021-01454-5

[91] Gokeler A, Benjaminse A, Welling W, Alferink M, Eppinga P, Otten B. The effects of attentional focus on jump

performance and knee joint kinematics in patients after ACL reconstruction. Physical Therapy in Sport. 2015;**16**:114-120. DOI: 10.1016/j.ptsp.2014.06.002

[92] Benjaminse A, Welling W, Otten B, Gokeler A. Novel methods of instruction in ACL injury prevention programs, a systematic review. Physical Therapy in Sport. 2015;**16**:176-186. DOI: 10.1016/j.ptsp.2014.06.003

[93] Gokeler A, Seil R, Kerkhoffs G, Verhagen E. A novel approach to enhance ACL injury prevention programs. Journal of Experimental Orthopaedics. 2018;**5**:22. DOI: 10.1186/s40634-018-0137-5

[94] Sadoghi P, von Keudell A, Vavken P. Effectiveness of anterior cruciate ligament injury prevention training programs. The Journal of Bone and Joint Surgery. American Volume. 2012;**94**:769-776. DOI: 10.2106/JBJS.K.00467

[95] Benjaminse A, Gokeler A, Dowling AV, Faigenbaum A, Ford KR, Hewett TE, et al. Optimization of the anterior cruciate ligament injury prevention paradigm: Novel feedback techniques to enhance motor learning and reduce injury risk. The Journal of Orthopaedic and Sports Physical Therapy. 2015;**45**:170-182. DOI: 10.2519/jospt.2015.4986

[96] Piccoli A, Rossettini G, Cecchetto S, Viceconti A, Ristori D, Turolla A, et al. Effect of attentional focus instructions on motor learning and performance of patients with central nervous system and musculoskeletal disorders: A systematic review. Journal of Functional Morphology and Kinesiology. 2018;**3**:40. DOI: 10.3390/jfmk3030040

[97] Blank R, Barnett AL, Cairney J, Green D, Kirby A, Polatajko H, et al. International clinical practice recommendations on the definition, diagnosis, assessment, intervention, and psychosocial aspects of developmental coordination disorder. Developmental Medicine and Child Neurology. 2019;**61**:242-285. DOI: 10.1111/dmcn.14132

[98] Gibbs J, Appleton J, Appleton R. Dyspraxia or developmental coordination disorder? Unravelling the enigma. Archives of Disease in Childhood. 2007;**92**:534-539. DOI: 10.1136/adc.2005.088054

[99] Smits-Engelsman B, Vinçon S, Blank R, Quadrado VH, Polatajko H, Wilson PH. Evaluating the evidence for motor-based interventions in developmental coordination disorder: A systematic review and meta-analysis. Research in Developmental Disabilities. 2018;**74**:72-102. DOI: 10.1016/j.ridd.2018.01.002

[100] Smits-Engelsman BC, Blank R, van der Kaay AC, Mosterd-van der Meijs R, Vlugt-van den Brand E, Polatajko HJ, et al. Efficacy of interventions to improve motor performance in children with developmental coordination disorder: A combined systematic review and meta-analysis. Developmental Medicine and Child Neurology. 2013;**55**:229-237. DOI: 10.1111/dmcn.12008

[101] Yu JJ, Burnett AF, Sit CH. Motor skill interventions in children with developmental coordination disorder: A systematic review and Meta-analysis. Archives of Physical Medicine and Rehabilitation. 2018;**99**:2076-2099. DOI: 10.1016/j.apmr.2017.12.009

[102] Lucas BR, Elliott EJ, Coggan S, Pinto RZ, Jirikowic T, McCoy SW, et al. Interventions to improve gross motor performance in children with neurodevelopmental disorders: A

meta-analysis. BMC Pediatrics. 2016;**16**:193. DOI: 10.1186/s12887-016-0731-6

[103] Visser J. Developmental coordination disorder: A review of research on subtypes and comorbidities. Human Movement Science. 2003;**22**:479-493. DOI: 10.1016/j.humov.2003.09.005

[104] Jarus T, Ghanouni P, Abel RL, Fomenoff SL, Lundberg J, Davidson S, et al. Effect of internal versus external focus of attention on implicit motor learning in children with developmental coordination disorder. Research in Developmental Disabilities. 2015;**37**:119-126. DOI: 10.1016/j.ridd.2014.11.009

[105] Watemberg N, Waiserberg N, Zuk L, Lerman-Sagie T. Developmental coordination disorder in children with attention-deficit-hyperactivity disorder and physical therapy intervention. Developmental Medicine and Child Neurology. 2007;**49**:920-925. DOI: 10.1111/j.1469-8749.2007.00920.x

[106] Psotta R, Abdollahipour R, Janura M. The effects of attentional focus instruction on the performance of a whole-body coordination task in children with developmental coordination disorder. Research in Developmental Disabilities. 2020;**101**:103654. DOI: 10.1016/j.ridd.2020.103654

[107] Li LL, Li YC, Chu CH, Pan CY, Chen FC. External focus of attention concurrently elicits optimal performance of suprapostural pole-holding task and postural stability in children with developmental coordination disorder. Neuroscience Letters. 2019;**703**:32-37. DOI: 10.1016/j.neulet.2019.03.011

Chapter 2

Potential Applications of Motor Imagery for Improving Standing Posture Balance in Rehabilitation

Shoya Fujikawa, Chihiro Ohsumi, Ryu Ushio, Kousuke Tamura, Shun Sawai, Ryosuke Yamamoto and Hideki Nakano

Abstract

Improving standing posture balance is an essential role of rehabilitation to prevent falls in the elderly and stroke victims. Recently, motor imagery has been reported to be an effective method to improve standing posture balance. Motor imagery is a simulation of a movement in the brain without actual movement. Motor imagery is believed to have a common neural basis with actual movement and is effective in reconstructing motor functions. Recently, it has also been shown that motor imagery can be enhanced through use in combination with neuromodulation techniques. In this chapter, motor imagery contributing to the improvement of standing postural balance and its combination with neuromodulation techniques are reviewed.

Keywords: motor imagery, kinesthetic imagery, visual imagery, standing balance, posture control, neuromodulation, neurofeedback, transcranial electrical stimulation, transcranial magnetic stimulation

1. Introduction

An important role of rehabilitation is to improve the standing postural balance of the elderly and stroke victims to prevent falls. Recently, motor imagery has been reported to effectively improve standing postural balance and facilitate the effects of neuromodulation techniques. This chapter outlines how motor imagery contributes to the improvement of standing postural balance and reviews how this method can be used in combination with neuromodulation techniques.

2. Motor imagery

Motor imagery is the simulation of motion in the brain without actual motion [1]. According to the PubMed database, 3853 articles on motor imagery were reviewed from 1979 to 2021, and the number is increasing every year. In addition, 1178 articles on rehabilitation using motor imagery were reviewed from 1999 to 2021, and the number of articles in this subtopic is also increasing, indicating that the application

IntechOpen

of motor imagery in rehabilitation has been attracting attention in recent years (**Figure 1**). In addition, motor imagery has a common neural basis with actual movement and is considered to be effective in reconstructing motor function. Therefore, clarification of brain activity during motor imagery will enhance the validity of motor function reconstruction by comparing it with brain activity during the actual exercise. In this section, we review the neural basis and mechanisms of motor imagery based on previous studies.

2.1 Brain function studies on motor imagery

In 1977, Ingvar and Philipson [2] introduced the first method for displaying the mean blood flow distribution in the brain as a two-dimensional color map in the study of brain function during motor imagery. They used this method to measure and compare regional cerebral blood flow at rest, during motor imagery, and during actual movement. Subjects performed a task in which they were asked to imagine a rhythmical clasping movement of the right hand during motor imagery and then perform a rhythmical movement of the right hand during actual movement. The measurement procedure in this study was the same for all subjects, with the resting state being measured first, followed by the motor imagery, and finally the actual exercise. The results showed that motor imagery increased blood flow in the entire frontal lobe, including the supraorbital region, as well as the parietal and temporal lobe regions. However, the actual movement of the right hand increased blood flow mainly in the central sulcus. Thus, the results of this study suggest that the centers of motor imagery are located in a different region of the cerebrum than the centers that control actual hand movements. However, medical science and technology have made

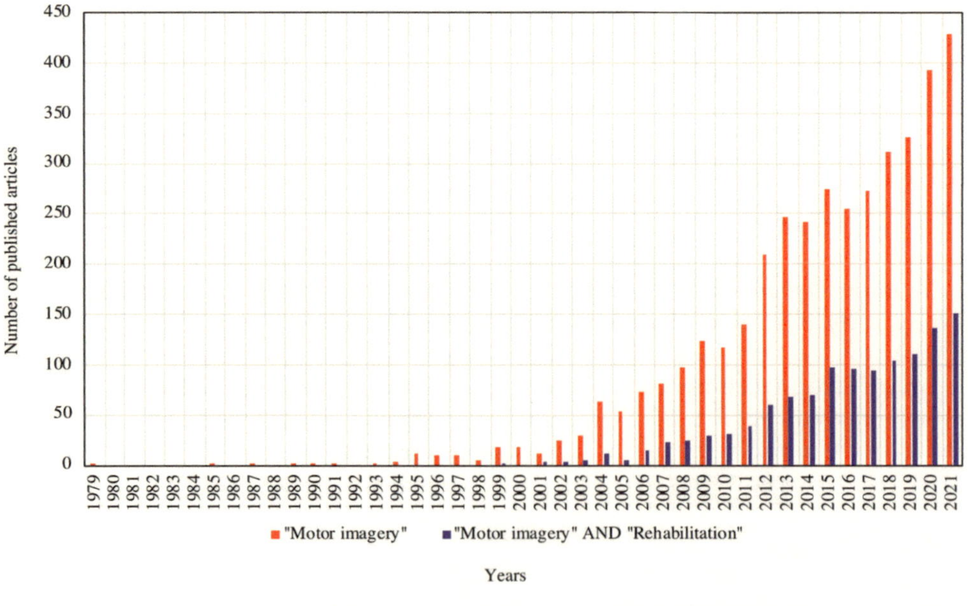

Figure 1.
Progression of the number of publications on motor imagery and the number of publications on motor imagery and rehabilitation. The red line shows the number of publications on motor imagery from 1977 to 2021. The blue line shows the number of publications on motor imagery and rehabilitation from 1999 to 2021. Data were collected from the PubMed database (https://pubmed.ncbi.nlm.nih.gov/) by online searches with the terms "motor imagery" for the red lines and "motor imagery" and "rehabilitation" for the blue lines.

obvious progress since 1977, and new techniques, such as functional magnetic resonance imaging (fMRI) [3] and positron emission tomography (PET) [4], have been used to detect brain activity. Moreover, Hétu et al. [5] performed an activation likelihood estimation (ALE) meta-analysis of 75 studies measuring brain activity during motor imagery using fMRI or PET reported up to 2011. They were the first to examine quantitative maps of structures activated during motor imagery. The results revealed that motor imagery depends on a network that includes motor-related areas, such as frontoparietal and subcortical structures. Therefore, studies from recent years have supported the view that motor imagery and actual movement share a common neural basis. In addition, a study from 2018 [6] that compared brain activity during motor imagery and actual movement in detail reported that there is effective connectivity between motor and cognitive networks. In that study, 20 healthy subjects were tested in a series of finger tapping trials, and electroencephalography (EEG) data throughout the task were validated using dynamic causal modeling. The results demonstrated effective connectivity between the dorsolateral prefrontal cortex (DLPFC) and secondary motor areas (M2), and between primary motor areas (M1) and M2, both during motor imagery and motor execution. Furthermore, DLPFC-premotor cortex (PMC) connectivity was more strongly activated during motor imagery than during actual movement. Additionally, PMC-supplementary motor areas (SMA) connectivity and M1-PMC connectivity were more strongly activated during motor imagery than during actual movement. Thus, in addition to supporting the recent view that motor imagery and actual movement share a common neural basis, the results of that study also suggest that although they share a common neural basis, they are distinct processes. In light of the above, reports on motor imagery are increasing annually, and subsequent studies are expected to elucidate brain activity during motor imagery.

2.2 Classification of motor imagery

Motor imagery can be divided into two types—muscular sensory imagery (KI) and visual imagery (VI). Because these methods of imagery differ, resulting in differing brain activity and training effects [7], the characteristics of each method must be understood to flexibly introduce motor imagery training in rehabilitation and elicit its effects. Guillot et al. [8] used fMRI to determine whether the neural networks formed by KI and VI are equivalent. In this study, 13 subjects were given a finger movement as a motor imagery task. The results of the comparison between KI and VI showed that movement-related structures and the inferior parietal lobule (IPL) were activated in KI, whereas the occipital lobule and superior parietal lobule (SPL) were mainly activated in VI. **Figure 2** shows the results of the evoked responses obtained for KI and VI during the 5 s of the test using a FASTRAK digitizer (Polhemus, Colchester, Vermont, USA), based on the neurophysiological data measured by the magnetoencephalography system. From the figure, it can be seen that KI results in outstanding PMC activity, while VI results in an activated occipital lobe. In addition, **Figure 3** shows the power spectra of brain activity measured by EEG for four activities—kinesthetic motor imagery (KMI), visual motor imagery (VMI), motor execution (ME), and visual observation (VO). Panel (a) shows that the normalized power of the KMI and VMI conditions was similar in the alpha and beta frequency bands. Panel (b) demonstrates that the neural networks were similar in KMI and ME due to their high connectivity to regions of interest (ROI) in the sensorimotor cortex. Furthermore, VMI and VO networks were similar, with a large number of networks distributed in the DLPFC and PMC. Moreover, Hétu et al. [5] reported in detail the brain regions

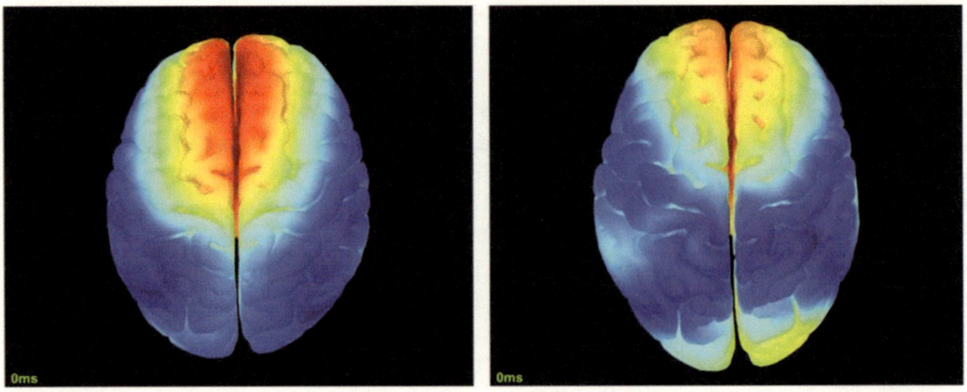

Figure 2.
Typical induced responses in KI and VI [9]. Right: induced response in KI. Left: induced response in VI.

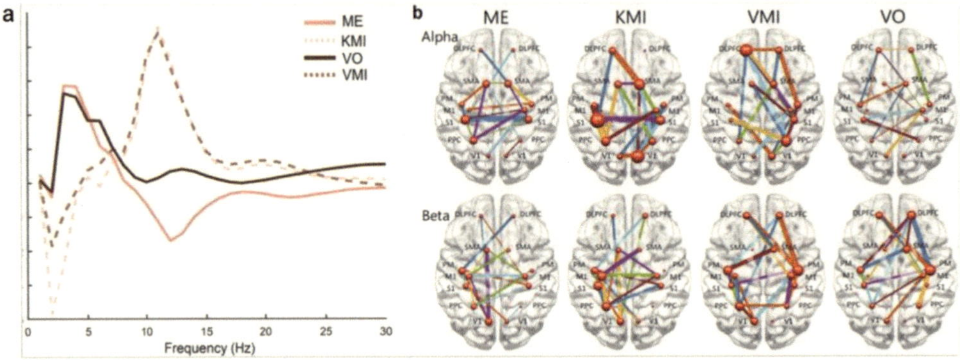

Figure 3.
Power spectra and connectivity in ME, KMI, VMI, and VO brain activity [10]. (a) Grand average power spectra of the four groups. Each line represents the grand average of the normalized power of each group with all seven subjects and ROIs. (b) The average of the maximum 20% connectivity in each of the four frequency bands. The line represents the functional connectivity calculated from the mutual information, and the thickness of the edge represents the strength of the connectivity. The node represents the location of the ROI, and the size of the node represents the connectivity with other ROIs.

that are consistently activated during KI and VI execution. KI showed consistent activation of the SMA, IPL, precentral gyrus (PcG), cerebellum (CB), left inferior frontal gyrus (IFG), supramarginal gyrus (SMG), temporal pole, putamen, anterior insula, right Rolandic operculum, angular gyrus, and pallidum. VI showed consistent activation of the bilateral SMA, left PcG, lingual gyrus, CB, light middle frontal gyrus (MFG), and postcentral gyrus (PocG). When KI and VI were combined, the left PcG, SMA, anterior insula, and bilateral putamen were consistently activated. Therefore, KI is employed during the execution of real movements, while VI is activated in the visual cortex, which processes visual information.

3. Motor imagery and standing postural balance

Improvement of standing postural balance consists of muscle strength [11, 12]; joint range of motion [13]; and somatosensory [14], visual [15], and brain function [16]. Moreover, standing postural balance and fall prevention are correlated, and it has been shown that control of lateral stability is significant for fall prevention interventions [17, 18]. Recently, motor imagery has been attracting attention as an intervention to improve balance function and the effects of motor imagery on standing postural balance have been reported in healthy subjects, the elderly, patients with stroke, and those with Parkinson's disease, among others. In this section, we review the effects of motor imagery on standing postural balance compared by subject based on previous studies.

3.1 Motor imagery and standing postural balance in healthy and elderly subjects

In a study on healthy subjects, Jahn et al. [19] examined the activation/deactivation patterns of each brain region during motor imagery using fMRI in imagery tasks of standing posture, walking, running, and supine posture. In this study, 13 healthy adults with an average age of 27.3 years performed the above-mentioned four motor imagery tasks for 20 s each in the supine position with closed eyes. The results showed that different activation/deactivation patterns were detected in the three conditions of standing, walking, and running, respectively. During motor imagery of the standing posture, the thalamus, basal ganglia, and cerebellar mediastinum were activated. During motor imagery of walking, the parahippocampal gyrus and cuneiform gyrus, occipital visual area, and CB were significantly activated. Moreover, during motor imagery of running, the cerebellar vermis and adjacent cerebellar hemispheres in the CB were activated six times more than during motor imagery in the standing and walking conditions, while the parahippocampal gyrus and cuneus gyrus were not activated compared to the walking condition. These results support the concept of hierarchical organization of posture and movement and suggest that motor imagery activates low-intensity CB activity that controls standing postural balance and the sensory-motor control through the thalamus and basal ganglia. In addition, a study has examined the effects of nonphysical training on standing postural balance from the perspective of brain activity [20]. The intervention involved 16 healthy adults with an average age of 27.5 years. The study was conducted under three conditions: (1) a combination of action observation and motor imagery in which the subjects watched a video of a balance task being performed, (2) simple action observation in which they watched a video, and (3) simple motor imagery in which they imagined walking with their eyes closed. Two balance tasks were performed under each condition: static standing and dynamic standing with internal and external perturbations, which were measured four times for static trials and four times for dynamic trials in a randomly determined order. The results showed that the intervention of motor imagery during the dynamic balance task predominantly activated the putamen, CB, SMA, and M1, and the combination of action observation and motor imagery activated the PMC in addition to the brain regions activated in motor imagery alone. However, intervention with action observation did not significantly activate these brain regions. In other words, this study suggests that motor imagery training may be effective in controlling standing posture in the medial and lateral directions.

In a study of older adults, Oh et al. [21] examined the potential for effective training adaptations for fall prevention by assessing static and dynamic balance and fear of falling in older adults who have a history of falls, before and after motor imagery training or task-oriented training. This study included 34 elderly subjects aged 65 years or older, randomly assigned to three groups: a motor imagery (11 subjects), task-oriented training (11 subjects), and a control group (12 subjects). In motor imagery training, the subjects sat in a sitting posture with their eyes closed during a 10-min relaxation period. Then, they imagined movements to protect themselves in the event of a fall for

20 min. In task-oriented training, balance training focusing on daily activities was conducted. The results showed that dynamic balance and fear of falling were significantly improved in the motor imagery group compared to the other two groups. Therefore, motor imagery training for the elderly and those without disease improved balance function, suggesting that it is highly effective as an intervention for fall prevention.

3.2 Motor imagery and standing postural balance in stroke patients

In 2005, a systematic review of seven databases on the effectiveness of motor imagery interventions in stroke patients [22] revealed a significant effect of motor imagery training in the Fugl-Meyer Stroke Assessment (FMA). In another study, a 30-minute motor imagery task of daily activities was performed on the paralyzed upper limbs, and changes in the cortex were verified by fMRI after 10 weeks of intervention [23]. This study revealed significant activation in the bilateral PMC and M1, as well as in the superior parietal lobe of the paralyzed side for flexion or extension movements of the wrist on the paralyzed side. These studies suggest that intervention with motor imagery training is effective for improving function in stroke patients.

In addition, a meta-analysis of balance function in stroke patients was performed in 2016 by extracting randomized controlled trials of motor imagery intervention for gait ability and balance in stroke patients from 12 electronic databases [24]. This study reported that intervention with motor imagery is effective in improving gait performance, but no statistical difference was found concerning balance function. According to Oostra et al. [25], poor motor imagery after stroke is associated with lesions of the left putamen, left ventral premotor cortex (PMv), and long association fibers connecting the parietooccipital region and the DLPFC. In other words, the effect of motor imagery is less clearly defined when the frontoparietal network is impaired. It has also been reported that the effect of motor imagery in stroke patients depends on their ability to maintain and manipulate information in working memory [26]. Moreover, the working memory involves the frontoparietal network [27], and it is highly likely that the basal ganglia and PMC have a strong influence on motor imagery. Additionally, the frontoparietal network has been reported to be the same brain region that is activated in actual movement [5]. Thus, a part of the frontoparietal network that is related to motor imagery as well as the actual movement was impaired, which affected the result that balance function was not significantly improved in the stroke patients. However, many studies have reported statistically significant effects on walking ability and upper limb function, suggesting that screening for motor imagery effectiveness based on lesion localization is necessary.

3.3 Motor imagery and standing postural balance in patients with Parkinson's disease

Parkinson's disease (PD) presents with movement [28], cognitive [29], and psychiatric symptoms [30]. PD can be clinically classified into a tremor-dominant subtype and a postural instability gait disorder subtype, and it has been reported that balance function is more impaired and the risk of falling is higher in the postural instability gait disorder subtype than in the tremor-dominant subtype [31, 32]. In addition, the severity of the postural instability gait disturbance is a useful indicator of PD severity and prognosis [33], suggesting that improvement in balance function and walking ability may be attributed to a favorable prognosis.

Motor imagery interventions for PD have been reported in many studies. For example, Thobois et al. used PET to compare the brain activity of normal subjects and immobilized PD subjects who imagined continuous hand movements [34]. The results showed that the prefrontal cortex, SMA, superior parietal lobe, IFG, and CB were activated during motor imagery in normal healthy subjects, while M1 activation was only observed during the dominant hand trials. Furthermore, in PD patients, motor imagery of the immobile hand showed a lack of activation in the contralateral primary somatosensory cortex and CB, persistent activation in the SMA, and bilateral activation in the superior parietal lobes. Based on these results, this study reports that PD patients with immobility show abnormal brain activation during motor imagery and that ideal brain activation depends on the state of the imagery hand.

Another symptom of PD is the altered timing of continuous movements. It has been shown that movement timing in internally generated continuous movements is selectively deficient, and the defects can lead to problems in movement planning [35]. This symptom may limit the conduct and potential effectiveness of motor imagery in rehabilitation for PD patients. Therefore, Heremans et al. validated the effects of a goal-directed motor imagery task using visual and auditory cues [36]. The results showed that the motor imagery task with visual cues significantly reduced bradykinesia. Moreover, the results suggest that the effectiveness of motor imagery for restoring function in PD patients can be enhanced by employing VI, while the effectiveness of KI is low. A study of VI intervention in PD patients examined the effects on standing postural balance and walking ability [37]. In this study, VO and motor imagery were administered as VI for 6 weeks. The results showed improved balance function and gait velocity in PD patients with postural instability and gait impairment. Thus, the addition of VI to standing postural balance training in PD patients promoted specific functional reorganization of brain regions involved in motor control and executive-attentional abilities, which is expected to have a long-term effect.

4. Neuromodulation techniques facilitated motor imagery effects

Motor imagery can be easily introduced into clinical practice because it can improve performance without special equipment. However, mental practice using motor imagery is limited in that the quality of the motor imagery being performed is not feedbacked to the subject [38], which causes individual differences in the motor imagery effects [39]. Neuromodulation technology has recently attracted attention as a method to solve this problem. Neuromodulation is a technique used to regulate the nervous system by electrical or scientific measures and is applied for many diseases [40]. Using this technology to provide feedback to the subject on the quality of motor imagery may be effective in improving movement performance. In this section, we review various neuromodulation techniques that facilitate motor imagery.

4.1 Combined motor imagery and neurofeedback

Neurofeedback is a noninvasive tool for purposeful modulation of human brain function that has the potential to dramatically impact neuroscience and clinical treatment of neuropsychiatric disorders [41]. Boe et al. [42] investigated whether the combined use of neurofeedback during motor imagery tasks could modulate brain activity. In this study, 18 healthy subjects (eight males, ten females, 24.7 ± 3.8 years old) were randomly assigned to a neurofeedback group or a control group. The motor imagery task was a KI activity in which the subject continuously pressed buttons with the ineffective hand. Neurofeedback was based on event-related synchronization/desynchronization (ERS/ERD) in the β-band of the sensorimotor cortex and was provided in real-time during motor imagery from a bar graph on a projector. The results showed that neurofeedback from bilateral sensory-motor cortices increased the contralateral pattern of brain activity associated with motor imagery with each successive session compared to the control group. Thus, this study suggests that the provision of neurofeedback provides significant information about motor imagery training and an opportunity for patients to modulate their own regional brain activation. In addition, neurofeedback approaches have a background of dependence on a single brain imaging modality such as EEG or fMRI. However, a study validated breaking away from this dependency system by reporting the effects of bimodal neurofeedback with simultaneous EEG and fMRI feedback [43]. In this study, the effects of unimodal EEG- and fMRI-neurofeedback were compared with those of bimodal EEG-fMRI-neurofeedback. The results showed that EEG-fMRI-neurofeedback significantly modulated activity in the movement domain compared to the two groups of short-peaked neurofeedback, and specific mechanisms and their additional value were found. Other studies have examined the effects of EEG-fMRI-neurofeedback on motor imagery, and all have shown that neurofeedback can modulate brain activity better than unimodal neurofeedback [44, 45]. In conclusion, neurofeedback during motor imagery can modulate brain activity and improve performance. Furthermore, incorporating multimodal techniques, such as bimodal neurofeedback instead of unimodal neurofeedback, may enhance the effects obtained from motor imagery.

4.2 Motor imagery and tES

Transcranial electrical stimulation (tES) aims to noninvasively modulate brain function by applying current from the current source [46]. Cranial electro-stimulation therapy (CET), cranial electrotherapy stimulation (CES), and transcranial pulsed current noise stimulation (tRNS) are several methods of tES used as clinical treatment [47]. Several previous studies have reported the use of tES, especially transcranial direct current stimulation (tDCS) and transcranial alternating current stimulation in combination with motor imagery. Moreover, Xie et al. [48] examined the effects of tES on brain activity during motor imagery. The results showed that ERD of μ and β rhythms during a motor imagery task was significantly enhanced by the combined use of tDCS with motor imagery. In addition, a study that examined the modulation of motor learning by transcranial alternating current stimulation [tACS] [49] suggested that 70 Hz tACS enhances motor learning ability by intermodulation activity in the β-wave band. Thus, tDCS and tACS are potential approaches to modulate brain activity during motor imagery and enhance effective functions to improve performance.

4.3 Motor imagery and rTMS

Transcranial magnetic stimulation (TMS) is a technique that noninvasively modulates brain activity through the induction of currents by rapidly changing magnetic field pulses [50]. In addition, by reviewing the literature through 2018, guidelines were established for treatment with repetitive transcranial magnetic stimulation (rTMS) in Europe in 2020. The guidelines established rTMS as a clinical treatment modality, although its efficacy has not reached Level A/B evidence.

Moreover, rTMS can be divided into high frequency (HF) and low frequency (LF) rTMS. LF rTMS decreases the excitability of the nonaffected hemisphere [51], while HF rTMS increases it [52].

Many previous studies in which motor imagery and rTMS were combined have verified the therapeutic effects on upper limb function in stroke victims [53, 54]. For example, Pan et al. [54] investigated the effects of motor imagery and LF rTMS on upper limb motor function during stroke rehabilitation. They applied 1 Hz rTMS to the M1 of the nonaffected hemisphere; 10 sessions of 30 min were performed during a two-week intervention period. The results showed that upper limb motor function was significantly improved in the group that received motor imagery and LF rTMS in the second and fourth weeks after the intervention compared to the control group (LF rTMS-only group). Moreover, a study in which motor imagery was combined with HF rTMS [55] also revealed a significant improvement in pre- and post-stimulation performance. These results suggest that rTMS can enhance the effects obtained from motor imagery in subjects such as stroke survivors. Finally, it was suggested that there is no difference between high and low rTMS frequencies in terms of performance improvement.

5. Conclusion

In this chapter, we outlined motor imagery effects that contribute to the improvement of standing postural balance and the effects that can result from use in combination with neuromodulation techniques. We further discussed the consequences for healthy subjects and those with illnesses. Recently, the view that motor imagery constitutes the same neural basis as actual movement is gaining ground, and the main effects of motor imagery in improving standing postural balance have been demonstrated. In addition, neuromodulation technology has the potential to improve the effects of motor imagery and is expected to further contribute to rehabilitation. Thus, the combination of neuromodulation techniques with motor imagery training will be significant in improving the quality of rehabilitation.

Acknowledgements

This work was supported by the Yuumi Memorial Foundation for Home Health Care and JSPS KAKENHI Grant Number JP20K11173.

Conflict of interest

The authors declare no conflict of interest.

Appendices and nomenclature

fMRI	functional magnetic resonance imaging
PET	positron emission tomography
ALE	activation likelihood estimation
DLPFC	dorsolateral prefrontal cortex

M1	primary motor areas
M2	secondary motor areas
PMC	premotor cortex
SMA	supplementary motor areas
KI	kinesthetic imagery
VI	visual imagery
IPL	inferior parietal lobule
SPL	superior parietal lobule
ME	motor execution
VO	visual observation
EEG	electroencephalography
ROI	regions of interest
PcG	precentral gyrus
CB	cerebellum
IFG	inferior frontal gyrus
SMG	supramarginal gyrus
MFG	middle frontal gyrus
PocG	postcentral gyrus
FMA	Fugl-Meyer Stroke Assessment
PMv	ventral premotor cortex
PD	Parkinson's disease
tES	transcranial electrical stimulation
CET	cranial electro stimulation therapy
CES	cranial electrotherapy stimulation
tPCS	transcranial pulsed current stimulation
tDCS	transcranial direct current stimulation
tACS	transcranial Alternating Current Stimulation
tRNS	transcranial Random Noise Stimulation
TMS	transcranial magnetic stimulation
rTMS	repetitive transcranial magnetic stimulation
HF	high frequency
LF	low frequency

Author details

Shoya Fujikawa[1], Chihiro Ohsumi[1], Ryu Ushio[1], Kousuke Tamura[1], Shun Sawai[2,3], Ryosuke Yamamoto[4] and Hideki Nakano[1,2*]

1 Faculty of Health Sciences, Neurorehabilitation Laboratory, Department of Physical Therapy, Kyoto Tachibana University, Kyoto, Japan

2 Neurorehabilitation Laboratory, Graduate School of Health Sciences, Kyoto Tachibana University, Kyoto, Japan

3 Department of Rehabilitation, Kyoto Kuno Hospital, Kyoto, Japan

4 Department of Rehabilitation, Tesseikai Neurosurgical Hospital, Osaka, Japan

*Address all correspondence to: nakano-h@tachibana-u.ac.jp

IntechOpen

© 2022 The Author(s). Licensee IntechOpen. This chapter is distributed under the terms of the Creative Commons Attribution License (http://creativecommons.org/licenses/by/3.0), which permits unrestricted use, distribution, and reproduction in any medium, provided the original work is properly cited. (cc) BY

References

[1] Jeannerod M. The representing brain. Neural correlates of motor intention and imagery. The Behavioral and Brain Sciences. 1994;**17**(2):187-202. DOI: 10.1017/s0140525x00034026

[2] Ingvar DH, Philipson L. Distribution of cerebral blood flow in the dominant hemisphere during motor ideation and motor performance. Annals of Neurology. 1997;**2**(3):230-237. DOI: 10.1002/ana.410020309

[3] Chen JE, Glover GH. Functional magnetic resonance imaging methods. Neuropsychology Review. 2015;**25**(3):289-313. DOI: 10.1007/s11065-015-9294-9

[4] Heurling K, Leuzy A, Jonasson M, Frick A, Zimmer ER, Nordberg A, et al. Quantitative positron emission tomography in brain research. Brain Research. 2017;**1670**:220-234. DOI: 10.1016/j.brainres.2017.06.022

[5] Hétu S, Grégoire M, Saimpont A, Coll MP, Eugène F, Michon PE, et al. The neural network of motor imagery: An ALE meta-analysis. Neuroscience and Biobehavioral Reviews. 2013;**37**(5):930-949. DOI: 10.1016/j.neubiorev.2013.03.017

[6] Kim YK, Park E, Lee A, Im CH, Kim YH. Changes in network connectivity during motor imagery and execution. PLoS One. 2018;**13**(1):e0190715. DOI: 10.1371/journal.pone.0190715

[7] Milton J, Small SL, Solodkin A. Imaging motor imagery: Methodological issues related to expertise. Methods. 2008;**45**(4):336-341. DOI: 10.1016/j.ymeth.2008.05.002

[8] Guillot A, Collet C, Nguyen VA, Malouin F, Richards C, Doyon J. Brain activity during visual versus kinesthetic imagery: An fMRI study. Human Brain Mapping. 2009;**30**(7):2157-2172. DOI: 10.1002/hbm.20658

[9] Chholak P, Niso G, Maksimenko VA, Kurkin SA, Frolov NS, Pitsik EN, et al. Visual and kinesthetic modes affect motor imagery classification in untrained subjects. Scientific Reports. 2019;**9**(1):1-12. DOI: 10.1038/s41598-019-46310-9

[10] Yang YJ, Jeon EJ, Kim JS, Chung CK. Characterization of kinesthetic motor imagery compared with visual motor imageries. Scientific Reports. 2021;**11**(1):3751. DOI: 10.1038/s41598-021-82241-0

[11] Tinetti ME, Kumar C. The patient who falls: "It's always a trade-off". Journal of the American Medical Association. 2010;**303**(3):258-266. DOI: 10.1001/jama.2009.2024

[12] Bijlsma AY, Pasma JH, Lambers D, Stijntjes M, Blauw GJ, Meskers CG, et al. Muscle strength rather than muscle mass is associated with standing balance in elderly outpatients. Journal of the American Medical Directors Association. 2013;**14**(7):493-498. DOI: 10.1016/j.jamda.2013.02.001

[13] Kim SG, Kim WS. Effect of Ankle Range of Motion (ROM) and lower-extremity muscle strength on static balance control ability in young adults: A regression analysis. Medical Science Monitor. 2018;**24**:3168-3175. DOI: 10.12659/MSM.908260

[14] Kars HJ, Hijmans JM, Geertzen JH, Zijlstra W. The effect of reduced somatosensation on standing balance: A

systematic review. Journal of Diabetes Science and Technology. 2009;**3**(4):931-943. DOI: 10.1177/193229680900300441

[15] Kennedy MW, Crowell CR, Striegel AD, Villano M, Schmiedeler JP. Relative efficacy of various strategies for visual feedback in standing balance activities. Experimental Brain Research. 2013;**230**(1):117-125

[16] Geurts AC, de Haart M, van Nes IJ, Duysens J. A review of standing balance recovery from stroke. Gait & Posture. 2005;**22**(3):267-281. DOI: 10.1007/s00221-013-3634-x

[17] Maki BE, Holliday PJ, Topper AK. A prospective study of postural balance and risk of falling in an ambulatory and independent elderly population. Journal of Gerontology. 1994;**49**(2):M72-M84. DOI: 10.1093/geronj/49.2.m72

[18] Piirtola M, Era P. Force platform measurements as predictors of falls among older people—A review. Gerontology. 2006;**52**(1):1-16. DOI: 10.1159/000089820

[19] Jahn K, Deutschländer A, Stephan T, Strupp M, Wiesmann M, Brandt T. Brain activation patterns during imagined stance and locomotion in functional magnetic resonance imaging. NeuroImage. 2004;**22**(4):1722-1731. DOI: 10.1016/j.neuroimage.2004.05.017

[20] Taube W, Mouthon M, Leukel C, Hoogewoud H-M, Annoni J-M, Keller M. Brain activity during observation and motor imagery of different balance tasks: An fMRI study. Cortex. 2015;**64**:102-114. DOI: 10.1016/j.cortex.2014.09.022

[21] Oh DS, Choi JD. Effects of motor imagery training on balance and gait in older adults: A randomized controlled pilot study. International Journal of Environmental Research and Public Health. 2021;**18**(2):650. DOI: 10.3390/ijerph18020650

[22] Zimmermann-Schlatter A, Schuster C, Puhan MA, Siekierka E, Steurer J. Efficacy of motor imagery in post-stroke rehabilitation: A systematic review. Journal of Neuroengineering and Rehabilitation. 2008;**5**:8. DOI: 10.1186/1743-0003-5-8

[23] Page SJ, Szaflarski JP, Eliassen JC, Pan H, Cramer SC. Cortical plasticity following motor skill learning during mental practice in stroke. Neurorehabilitation and Neural Repair. 2009;**23**(4):382-388. DOI: 10.1177/1545968308326427

[24] Li RQ, Li ZM, Tan JY, Chen GL, Lin WY. Effects of motor imagery on walking function and balance in patients after stroke: A quantitative synthesis of randomized controlled trials. Complementary Therapies in Clinical Practice. 2017;**28**:75-84. DOI: 10.1016/j.ctcp.2017.05.009

[25] Oostra KM, Van Bladel A, Vanhoonacker AC, Vingerhoets G. Damage to fronto-parietal networks impairs motor imagery ability after stroke: A voxel-based lesion symptom mapping study. Frontiers in Behavioral Neuroscience. 2016;**10**:5. DOI: 10.3389/fnbeh.2016.00005

[26] Malouin F, Belleville S, Richards CL, Desrosiers J, Doyon J. Working memory and mental practice outcomes after stroke. Archives of Physical Medicine and Rehabilitation. 2004;**85**(2):177-183. DOI: 10.1016/s0003-9993(03)00771-8

[27] Smith R, Lane RD, Alkozei A, et al. Maintaining the feelings of others in working memory is associated with activation of the left anterior insula and left frontal-parietal control network. Social Cognitive and Affective

Neuroscience. 2017;**12**(5):848-860. DOI: 10.1093/scan/nsx011

[28] Wu T, Hallett M, Chan P. Motor automaticity in Parkinson's disease. Neurobiology of Disease. 2015;**82**:226-234. DOI: 10.1016/j.nbd.2015.06.014

[29] Leverenz JB, Quinn JF, Zabetian C, Zhang J, Montine KS, Montine TJ. Cognitive impairment and dementia in patients with Parkinson disease. Current Topics in Medicinal Chemistry. 2009;**9**(10):903-912

[30] Zuo LJ, Yu SY, Hu Y, et al. Serotonergic dysfunctions and abnormal iron metabolism: Relevant to mental fatigue of Parkinson disease. Scientific Reports. 2016;**6**(1):19. DOI: 10.1038/s41598-016-0018-z

[31] Herman T, Weiss A, Brozgol M, Giladi N, Hausdorff JM. Gait and balance in Parkinson's disease subtypes: Objective measures and classification considerations. Journal of Neurology. 2014;**261**(12):2401-2410. DOI: 10.1007/s00415-014-7513-6

[32] Vervoort G, Bengevoord A, Nackaerts E, Heremans E, Vandenberghe W, Nieuwboer A. Distal motor deficit contributions to postural instability and gait disorder in Parkinson's disease. Behavioural Brain Research. 2015;**287**:1-7. DOI: 10.1016/j.bbr.2015.03.026

[33] van der Heeden JF, Marinus J, Martinez-Martin P, Rodriguez-Blazquez C, Geraedts VJ, van Hilten JJ. Postural instability and gait are associated with severity and prognosis of Parkinson disease. Neurology. 2016;**86**(24):2243-2250. DOI: 10.1212/WNL.0000000000002768

[34] Thobois S, Dominey PF, Decety J, Pollak PP, Gregoire MC, Le Bars PD, et al. Motor imagery in normal subjects and in asymmetrical Parkinson's disease: A PET study. Neurology. 2000;**55**(7):996-1002. DOI: 10.1212/wnl.55.7.996

[35] Avanzino L, Pelosin E, Martino D, Abbruzzese G. Motor timing deficits in sequential movements in Parkinson disease are related to action planning: A motor imagery study. PLoS One. 2013;**8**(9):e75454. DOI: 10.1371/journal.pone.0075454

[36] Heremans E, Nieuwboer A, Feys P, Vercruysse S, Vandenberghe W, Sharma N, et al. External cueing improves motor imagery quality in patients with Parkinson disease. Neurorehabilitation and Neural Repair. 2012;**26**(1):27-35. DOI: 10.1177/1545968311411055

[37] Sarasso E, Agosta F, Piramide N, Gardoni A, Canu E, Leocadi M, et al. Action observation and motor imagery improve dual task in parkinson's disease: A clinical/fMRI Study. Movement Disorders. 2021;**36**(11):2569-2582. DOI: 10.1002/mds.28717

[38] Bai O, Huang D, Fei DY, Kunz R. Effect of real-time cortical feedback in motor imagery-based mental practice training. NeuroRehabilitation. 2014;**34**(2):355-363. DOI: 10.3233/NRE-131039

[39] van der Meulen M, Allali G, Rieger SW, Assal F, Vuilleumier P. The influence of individual motor imagery ability on cerebral recruitment during gait imagery. Human Brain Mapping. 2014;**35**(2):455-470. DOI: 10.1002/hbm.22192

[40] Henderson JM, Federici T, Boulis N. Optogenetic neuromodulation. Neurosurgery. 2009;**64**(5):796-804. DOI: 10.1227/01.NEU.0000339171.87593.6A

[41] Hampson M, Ruiz S, Ushiba J. Neurofeedback. Neuroimage. 2020;**218**:116473. DOI: 10.1016/j.neuroimage.2019.116473

[42] Boe S, Gionfriddo A, Kraeutner S, Tremblay A, Little G, Bardouille T. Laterality of brain activity during motor imagery is modulated by the provision of source level neurofeedback. NeuroImage. 2014;**101**:159-167. DOI: 10.1016/j.neuroimage.2014.06.066

[43] Perronnet L, Lécuyer A, Mano M, Bannier E, Lotte F, Clerc M, et al. Unimodal versus bimodal EEG-fMRI neurofeedback of a motor imagery task. Frontiers in Human Neuroscience. 2017;**11**:193. DOI: 10.3389/fnhum.2017.00193

[44] Lioi G, Cury C, Perronnet L, Mano M, Bannier E, Lécuyer A, et al. Simultaneous EEG-fMRI during a neurofeedback task, a brain imaging dataset for multimodal data integration. Science Data. 2020;**7**(1):173. DOI: 10.1038/s41597-020-0498-3

[45] Zich C, Debener S, Kranczioch C, Bleichner MG, Gutberlet I, De Vos M. Real-time EEG feedback during simultaneous EEG-fMRI identifies the cortical signature of motor imagery. NeuroImage. 2015;**114**:438-447. DOI: 10.1016/j.neuroimage.2015.04.020

[46] Bikson M, Esmaeilpour Z, Adair D, Kronberg G, Tyler WJ, Antal A, et al. Transcranial electrical stimulation nomenclature. Brain Stimulation. 2019;**12**(6):1349-1366. DOI: 10.1016/j.brs.2019.07.010

[47] Guleyupoglu B, Schestatsky P, Edwards D, Fregni F, Bikson M. Classification of methods in transcranial electrical stimulation (tES) and evolving strategy from historical approaches to contemporary innovations. Journal of Neuroscience Methods. 2013;**219**(2):297-311. DOI: 10.1016/j.jneumeth.2013.07.016

[48] Xie J, Peng M, Lu J, Xiao C, Zong X, Wang M, et al. Enhancement of event-related desynchronization in motor imagery based on transcranial electrical stimulation. Frontiers in Human Neuroscience. 2021;**15**:635351. DOI: 10.3389/fnhum.2021.635351

[49] Sugata H, Yagi K, Yazawa S, Nagase Y, Tsuruta K, Ikeda T, et al. Modulation of motor learning capacity by transcranial alternating current stimulation. Neuroscience. 2018;**391**:131-139. DOI: 10.1016/j.neuroscience.2018.09.013

[50] Aceves-Serrano L, Neva JL, Doudet DJ. Insight into the effects of clinical repetitive transcranial magnetic stimulation on the brain from positron emission tomography and magnetic resonance imaging studies: A narrative review. Frontiers in Neuroscience. 2022;**16**:787403. DOI: 10.3389/fnins.2022.787403

[51] Du J, Yang F, Hu J, Hu J, Xu Q, Cong N, et al. Effects of high- and low-frequency repetitive transcranial magnetic stimulation on motor recovery in early stroke patients: Evidence from a randomized controlled trial with clinical, neurophysiological and functional imaging assessments. Neuroimage Clinical. 2019;**21**:101620. DOI: 10.1016/j.nicl.2018.101620

[52] Guo Z, Jin Y, Bai X, Jiang B, He L, McClure MA, et al. Distinction of high- and low-frequency repetitive transcranial magnetic stimulation on the functional reorganization of the motor network in stroke patients. Neural Plasticity. 2021;**2021**:8873221. DOI: 10.1155/2021/8873221

[53] Kang JH, Kim MW, Park KH, Choi YA. The effects of additional electrical stimulation combined with repetitive transcranial magnetic stimulation and motor imagery on upper extremity motor recovery in the subacute period after stroke: A preliminary study. Medicine (Baltimore). 2021;**100**(35):e27170. DOI: 10.1097/MD.0000000000027170

[54] Pan W, Wang P, Song X, Sun X, Xie Q. The effects of combined low frequency repetitive transcranial magnetic stimulation and motor imagery on upper extremity motor recovery following stroke. Frontiers in Neurology. 2019;**10**:96. DOI: 10.3389/fneur.2019.00096

[55] Jia T, Mo L, Li C, Liu A, Li Z, Ji L. 5 Hz rTMS improves motor-imagery based BCI classification performance. Annual International Conference of the IEEE Engineering in Medicine and Biology Society. 2021;**2021**:6116-6120. DOI: 10.1109/EMBC46164.2021.9630102

Chapter 3

Clinical Application of Repetitive Peripheral Magnetic Stimulation in Rehabilitation

Ryu Ushio, Kousuke Tamura, Shoya Fujikawa, Chihiro Ohsumi, Shun Sawai, Ryosuke Yamamoto and Hideki Nakano

Abstract

Repetitive peripheral magnetic stimulation (rPMS) is a noninvasive method involving the repetitive magnetic stimulation of peripheral nerves and muscles. Recently, its potential as a new neuromodulation technique for sensory motor disorders has been recognized. Its advantages include less pain than with electrical stimulation and that neuromuscular stimulation can be performed over clothing. These advantages make it a practical and straightforward adjunct tool widely used in clinical practice. In particular, the combination of rPMS and general rehabilitation reportedly promotes functional improvement in stroke patients with difficult involuntary contractions. This chapter reviews rPMS and its potential clinical applications in rehabilitation.

Keywords: repetitive peripheral magnetic stimulation, motor imagery, muscle strengthening, spasticity, stroke, motor recovery, rehabilitation, physical therapy

1. Introduction

Magnetic stimulation is the application of "electrode-free electrical stimulation" using induced current from a pulsed magnetic field. The magnetic field generated by the stimulation coil induces an electromagnetic-induced overcurrent in the body that resultantly depolarizes nerves and muscles' cell membranes, thereby stimulating the brain, nerves, and muscles. Repetitive peripheral magnetic stimulation (rPMS) is applied as a treatment method that noninvasively delivers repetitive magnetic stimulation to peripheral nerves and muscles. It has attracted attention as a new means of rehabilitation, especially for sensory and motor disorders [1].

To date, neuromuscular electrical stimulation (NMES) has been widely used as a similar tool. NMES is an electrical stimulation therapy primarily performed to improve motor function, such as suppressing muscle hypertonia associated with upper-motor neuron damage, preventing and improving muscle atrophy associated with peripheral neuropathy, and increasing muscle strength. However, this therapy is associated with pain and discomfort caused by electrical stimulation. Compared with NMES, rPMS does not cause discomfort due to pain and can stimulate deep muscles [2]. NMES evokes cutaneous receptors and may generate noisy signals, whereas rPMS generates intrinsic receptive information during muscle contraction that affects brain reversibility [3].

Furthermore, rPMS does not require the application of electrodes and can be stimulated over clothing. Similar to NMES, however, rPMS is contraindicated for pacemakers and implantable medical devices. In addition, rPMS is larger in size and more expensive than NMES, making its widespread use a challenge. However, rPMS is expected to improve functional recovery in stroke patients because of its ability to safely stimulate deeper layers and improve muscle areas without pain [4].

2. rPMS studies in healthy subjects

2.1 Physiological changes in rPMS

rPMS can improve motor function in central nervous system (CNS) diseases. How, then, would the induction of CNS plasticity be altered by the parameters of rPMS? Nito et al. [5] studied the effects of rPMS on wrist extensor muscles in terms of neuroplasticity and motor performance in 26 healthy subjects (HS). Motor-evoked potential (MEP), intracortical inhibition (ICI), intracortical facilitation (ICF), M-wave, and Hoffman reflex were measured before and after the application of rPMS, and the effects of rPMS on wrist extensor movements were examined.

First, rPMS was applied to the wrist extensor muscles at different frequencies (50, 25, and 10 Hz), with the total number of stimuli set constant to examine the physical effects of stimulus frequency. MEPs of the wrist extensors increased significantly with rPMS at 50 and 25 Hz but remained unchanged at 10 Hz. In the next experiment, in which the number of stimuli was increased and the time required to induce plasticity was examined, at least 15 minutes of rPMS were required for 50- and 25-Hz rPMS. Based on these parameters, the sustained effect of 50- or 25-Hz rPMS was evaluated after 15 minutes of rPMS. Significant increases in MEP were observed up to 60 minutes after 50- and 25-Hz rPMS were administered. Similarly, attenuation of ICI and enhancement of ICF were also observed.

In addition, the maximal M-wave and Hoffman reflex were unchanged, suggesting that the imposition of rPMS does not directly stimulate the centrifugal nerves and excite the muscles but that the increase in MEP is caused by the plastic changes in the motor cortex. In addition, an increase in force and EMG during wrist extension movements was observed after the application of rPMS at 50 and 25 Hz. These results suggest that the application of rPMS at 25 Hz or higher for 15 minutes can increase cortical excitability at the irradiated site and improve motor output from the motor cortex, rather than changing the excitability of the spinal cord circuitry.

Recent studies have also reported the effects of rPMS in combination with noninvasive brain stimulation techniques and on regions other than the periphery. Kumru et al. [6] examined the effects of paired associative stimulation (PAS), in which paired stimuli of repetitive transcranial magnetic stimulation (rTMS) and rPMS are repeatedly applied. PAS is an effective method to induce plasticity in the human motor cortex. Three stimulus conditions were applied to 11 HS for 10 minutes each. In the rPMS alone condition, rPMS at 10 Hz was applied to the extensor carpi radialis (ECR) five times every 10 seconds for 60 trials. In the rTMS alone condition, rTMS was applied to the contralateral primary motor cortex region of the ECR at a frequency of 0.1 Hz (60 stimuli) and an intensity of 120% of the ECR threshold. In the PAS condition, rPMS and rTMS described above were performed with paired stimuli. The results showed that the PAS condition increased MEP amplitude and decreased ICI in the ECR. This suggests that PAS stimulation effectively increases corticospinal tract excitability and decreases ICI. Krause et al. [7] studied the effects of repetitive magnetic stimulation (rMS) to the right cervical nerve root (C7/C8) on corticospinal excitability in HS. The right cervical nerve root (C7/C8) innervating the test muscle, the right first dorsal interosseous muscle, was stimulated at a frequency of 20 Hz for 10 seconds with an intensity of 120% of resting motor threshold for a total of 10 trials. The results showed that rMS caused a significantly longer cortical silent period, increased ICI, and increased MEP amplitude. These changes were not confirmed contralaterally. This study confirmed that rMS increased MEP amplitude in the right first dorsal interosseous muscle without altering the left dorsal interosseous muscle. These results indicate that rMS affects motor cortex excitability similar to electrical stimulation; this suggests that rMS is applicable in spastic and central paraplegia rehabilitation.

As described above, physiological changes in rPMS have been reported in HS, and based on these studies, various clinical application studies have been conducted in the recent years.

2.2 Changes in rPMS and motor imagery in combination

Motor imagery (MI) is the simulation of movement in the brain without actual movement and is widely used in clinical practice as a tool for evaluation and treatment. Recently, the combined effects of MI and rPMS have been reported.

Asao et al. [8] examined the effects of rPMS combined with MI (rPMS+MI) on corticospinal excitability. The rPMS+MI condition and rPMS alone condition were performed on HS. In the rPMS+MI condition, rPMS was administered simultaneously with a cue for a MI task of dorsiflexion of the right wrist joint. The test muscle was the right ECR. The rPMS frequency was 25 Hz, stimulus duration was 2 s, and stimulus intensity was 1.5 times the motor threshold. In the rPMS alone condition, rPMS was administered under the same stimulation conditions as in the rPMS+MI condition. The results showed that the pre- and post-stimulus MEP ratios were more significant in the rPMS+MI condition than in the rPMS alone-intense condition, which was associated with Movement Imagery Questionnaire-Revised scores. This study suggests that an intervention combining rPMS and MI can induce more corticospinal excitation than rPMS alone.

The studies above did not clarify the effective length of intervention period for the combination of rPMS and MI to promote corticospinal excitability. Therefore, the time course changes in corticospinal excitability when rPMS and MI are used in combination have been examined [9]. rPMS alone, MI alone, and rPMS and MI combination conditions have been performed on HS. In the rPMS alone and rPMS+MI conditions, the ECR was stimulated with rPMS at 25 Hz for 2 seconds at a stimulus intensity of 1.5 times the motor threshold. In addition, the MI and rPMS+MI groups were asked to perform MI of wrist dorsiflexion for 2 seconds.

Consequently, the MEP amplitude increase of the ECR in the rPMS+MI group was observed after 10 minutes. In addition, the MEP amplitude after 20 minutes was more significant in the rPMS+MI group than in the rPMS alone group. This study suggests that the combination of rPMS and MI over 10 minutes increases corticospinal excitation and that the combined effect is more significant than rPMS alone. Overall, the combination of rPMS and MI may induce plasticity in the CNS and promote motor function recovery.

3. Clinical applications of rPMS

3.1 Muscle-strengthening effects of rPMS

One of the clinical applications of rPMS is its muscle-strengthening effect. It has been reported that rPMS promotes muscle strengthening in animals and humans without causing pain.

Yang et al. [10] investigated the effects of neuromuscular magnetic stimulation (NMMS) on strength, cross-sectional area, and thickness of the quadriceps muscle in HS. NMMS was performed on the quadriceps femoris muscle at a frequency of 10 Hz and at the maximum tolerable intensity that could be tolerated for 15 minutes, thrice weekly for 5 weeks. The results showed that maximal isometric torque and mean peak torque increased significantly after intervention, but there was no change in cross-sectional area or thickness. This study suggests that NMMS effectively trains large or skeletal muscles such as the quadriceps.

Stolting et al. [11] showed that magnetic stimulation of a mouse muscle injury model caused post-traumatic muscle hypertrophy, but the effects of rPMS on human subjects remained unclear. Therefore, Hirono et al. [12] examined the acute changes in skeletal muscle thickness induced by rPMS after low-intensity exercise for clinical application of rPMS. rPMS was applied to the vastus lateralis muscle at the maximum intensity of the rPMS device after an HS performed three sets of 10 isometric knee extension exercises at 30% of maximum muscle strength. The results showed that the muscle thickness of the rectus femoris and vastus lateralis muscles after exercise increased over baseline values, with significant increases only in the vastus lateralis after rPMS. This study suggests that post-exercise rPMS induces muscle expansion *via* repetitive muscle contractions. Acute changes such as skeletal muscle expansion that occur immediately after exercise also reportedly play a significant role in subsequent muscle hypertrophy [13, 14].

rPMS has the advantage of not causing pain and has been used in clinical practice with the expectation of functional recovery in some cases. Beck et al. [15] studied the effect of early intervention with rPMS on the vastus lateralis muscle after hip replacement surgery. The subjects were patients who underwent hip replacement after a proximal femur fracture. The experimental group received 10 Hz rPMS on the vastus lateralis muscle for 15 sessions daily, five times weekly for 3 weeks, whereas the control group received sham stimulation. The results showed that the root-mean-square value of the electromyogram during the maximum voluntary contraction of the vastus lateralis muscle after rPMS was significantly improved. Tandem rise time and normal walking speed in the rPMS group also improved. This study suggests that early intervention with rPMS on the lateral vastus muscle after hip arthroplasty improves muscle strength, standing balance, and gait function. This study also indicates that rPMS can be applied to patients with pain and wounds and is expected to be widely applied in clinical practice in the future.

As described above, rPMS, which promotes muscle strengthening without causing pain, has excellent potential for clinical applications.

3.2 Application of rPMS in stroke rehabilitation

Post-stroke hemiplegia occurs in more than 85% of individuals and 55–75% have residual upper limb dysfunction [16]. After stroke, the recovery rate to a practical level is approximately 60% for lower limb function and approximately 20% for upper limb function [17]. The effectiveness of rehabilitation and physical therapy for stroke has been reported in many cases. In this context, the effectiveness of rPMS for stroke has been reported in recent years.

rPMS is a noninvasive method of activating peripheral nerves at the stimulation site and improving muscle strength and has the advantage of being performed without causing pain. Jiang et al. [18] applied rPMS in the early subacute phase of stroke and studied its effect on severe upper limb disability. In the intervention group, rPMS of 20 Hz, totaling 2400 pulses, was applied daily for 2 weeks to the triceps brachii and extensor digitorum brevis muscles. The results showed that the rPMS group showed significant improvements in the upper limb, Barthel Index, upper limb muscle strength, and root mean square on the Fugl-Meyer Assessment compared with those in the control group. This study demonstrates that rPMS for the upper extremity after stroke improves upper extremity function and muscle strength.

Fernandez-Lobera et al. [19] studied the efficacy of rPMS as a tool to assess wrist spasticity in stroke patients. The subjects were HS, acute stroke patients without spasticity (AS), and chronic stroke patients with spasticity (CS). Spasticity was assessed by calculating the index of movement restriction (iMR) from the difference between the maximum passive movement range of the wrist joint and the evoked movement range by rPMS. The stimulation intensity of rPMS was set at 70% of the maximum output of the stimulator, frequency at 25 Hz, and stimulation duration at 2 seconds. The results showed that the amplitude, velocity, and acceleration of rPMS-induced movements were reduced in the CS compared with those in the HS and AS. The iMR values were 2.8 for HS, 13.0 for AS, and 59.2 for CS, with CS having the highest iMR value. Furthermore, the iMR value for CS decreased to 41.1 after treatment with botulinum neurotoxin.

Shoulder joint subluxation is one of the many complications following stroke and is an inhibitor of motor function recovery [20]. In particular, shoulder joint subluxation causes pain in the shoulder joint and has a significant impact on activities of daily living. Therefore, Fujimura et al. [21] investigated the effect of rPMS on shoulder joint dislocation caused by stroke. The subjects were patients who presented with shoulder joint subluxation after stroke. rPMS was performed repetitively on the supraspinatus, posterior deltoid, and infraspinatus muscles. Stimulation intensity was the maximum tolerable intensity and was performed at 30 Hz for 2 seconds for 100 sessions. Results showed that the acromion-humerus interval was significantly reduced after treatment. That shoulder joint pain, shoulder abduction range of motion, and upper extremity scores on the Fugl-Meyer Assessment also improved. This study demonstrates that rPMS for post-stroke shoulder dislocation decreases the degree of shoulder subluxation and pain and improves upper extremity motor function.

Krewer et al. [22] examined the short- and long-term effects of rPMS on spasticity and motor function in stroke patients. rPMS involved a total of 5000 stimuli at 25 Hz and a stimulus intensity of 110% of the resting motor threshold. Stimulation was applied to the extensor and flexor muscles of the upper arm and forearm twice daily for 2 weeks. Results showed short-term effects on wrist flexor spasticity (immediately after the intervention) and long-term effects on elbow extensor spasticity (2 weeks after the intervention) in the rPMS group. In addition, the rPMS group showed an improvement in sensory function. This study demonstrates that rPMS reduces spasticity and improves sensory function in stroke patients in both short and long terms.

Kinoshita et al. [23] investigated the effects of rPMS on the lower limb of chronic stroke patients on gait function. The subjects were stroke patients with lower limb hemiplegia and gait disturbance. The stimulation sites of rPMS were the gluteus maximus, vastus medialis, hamstrings, quadriceps, gastrocnemius, and soleus muscles of the paralyzed lower limb. rPMS was performed twice daily for 15 days at a frequency of 20 Hz for 3 s, 4800 pulses, and a stimulus intensity of 110% of the motor threshold. The results showed that walking speed, walking ability, and balance ability were significantly improved after the intervention. This study suggests that rPMS effectively restores gait function in stroke patients with gait disturbance.

Beaulieu et al. [24] studied the effect of rPMS on lower limb dysfunction in chronic stroke. The stimulation site of rPMS was the anterior tibialis muscle of the paralyzed lower extremity. rPMS was performed at a theta-burst frequency (three 50 Hz pulses each, delivered in 5-Hz bursts) for 190 s at 42% of maximum stimulation intensity. The results showed that the rPMS group increased ankle dorsiflexion range of motion and maximum isometric muscle strength after the intervention and decreased resistance to ankle flexor stretch. The results also suggested that these changes are related to residual corticospinal tracts. This study demonstrates that rPMS improves lower limb dysfunction in chronic stroke patients.

In conclusion, rPMS improves upper and lower limb dysfunction in stroke patients. Therefore, we believe that rPMS is a highly effective tool for evaluation and treatment in stroke rehabilitation.

4. Conclusion

This chapter outlines the physiological changes, combined effects of MI, muscle strengthening, and effects on stroke patients in rPMS. The rPMS parameters used in studies are listed in **Tables 1** and **2**. rPMS has attracted attention as a new neuromodulation technique that can noninvasively deliver repetitive magnetic stimulation

	Stimulation site	Stimulation frequency	Stimulation intensity
Nito et al. [5]	Wrist extensor muscles	50 Hz, 25 Hz, 10 Hz	120% of the motor threshold
Kumru et al. [6]	Extensore carpi radialis muscle	rPMS: 10 Hz rTMS: 0.1 Hz	rPMS: 70% of motor threshold rTMS: 120% of motor threshold
Krause et al. [7]	Cervical nerve roots (C7/C8) (First dorsal interosseous)	20 Hz	120% of motor threshold
Asao et al. [8]	Extensore carpi radialis muscle	25 Hz	150% of motor threshold
Asao et al. [9]	Extensore carpi radialis muscle	25 Hz	150% of motor threshold
Yang et al. [10]	Quadriceps muscle	10 Hz	Maximum tolerable intensity
Hirono et al. [12]	Vastus lateralis muscle	50 Hz	Maximum intensity of the device

Table 1.
rPMS parameters in basic research on healthy subjects.

	Patients	Stimulation site	Stimulation frequency	Stimulation intensity
Beck et al. [15]	After hip replacement surgery	Vastus lateralis muscle	10 Hz	Level where the visible movement of the knee is triggered
Jiang et al. [18]	Early subacute stroke	Triceps brachii and extensor digitorum muscles	20 Hz	Triceps brachii muscle: Intensity to induce 30° of elbow extension Extensor digitorum muscle: Intensity to induce 45° of wrist extension
Fernandez-Lobera et al. [19]	Acute stroke without/with spasticity	Wrist extensor muscles	25 Hz	70% of the maximum stimulator power
Fujimura et al. [21]	Shoulder subluxations caused by stroke	Supraspinatus and posterior deltoid/ infraspinatus muscles	30 Hz	Intensity until patients indicates that any further increase would become uncomfortable
Krewer et al. [22]	Severe hemiparesis and mild to moderate spasticity resulting from a stroke or a traumatic brain injury	Extensors and flexors of the upper and lower arm.	25 Hz	110% of motor threshold
Kinoshita et al. [23]	Hemorrhagic stroke with lower limb hemiparesis and gait disturbance	Gluteus maximus muscle, gluteus medius, hamstring muscle, musculus quadriceps femoris, gastrocnemius, soleus	20 Hz	110% of motor threshold
Beaulieu et al. [24]	Chronic stroke	Tibialis anterior muscle	Theta-burst frequency (5-Hz bursts of three 50 Hz pulses each)	42% of the maximal stimulator output

Table 2.
rPMS parameters in clinical research.

to peripheral nerves and muscles using induced current from a pulsed magnetic field. Unlike NMES, rPMS is painless and has excellent potential for application in clinical settings. In particular, many clinical studies for stroke rehabilitation have been reported in recent years. Further development of rPMS research is expected, including its effectiveness when combined with other therapies and its integration with technology.

Acknowledgements

This work was supported by the Yuumi Memorial Foundation for Home Health Care and JSPS KAKENHI Grant Number JP20K11173.

Conflict of interest

The authors declare no conflict of interest.

Appendices and nomenclature

rPMS:	repetitive peripheral magnetic stimulation
NMES:	neuromuscular electrical stimulation
MEP:	motor-evoked potential
rTMS:	repetitive transcranial magnetic stimulation
PAS:	paired associative stimulation
ECR:	extensor carpi radialis
rMS:	repetitive magnetic stimulation
ICI:	intracortical inhibition
MI:	motor imagery
NMMS:	neuromuscular magnetic stimulation
HS:	healthy subjects
AS:	acute stroke patients without spasticity
CS:	chronic stroke patients with spasticity
iMR:	index of movement restriction

Author details

Ryu Ushio[1], Kousuke Tamura[1], Shoya Fujikawa[1], Chihiro Ohsumi[1], Shun Sawai[2,3], Ryosuke Yamamoto[4] and Hideki Nakano[1,2*]

1 Faculty of Health Sciences, Neurorehabilitation Laboratory, Department of Physical Therapy, Kyoto Tachibana University, Kyoto, Japan

2 Neurorehabilitation Laboratory, Graduate School of Health Sciences, Kyoto Tachibana University, Kyoto, Japan

3 Department of Rehabilitation, Kuno Hospital, Kyoto, Japan

4 Department of Rehabilitation, Tesseikai Neurosurgical Hospital, Osaka, Japan

*Address all correspondence to: nakano-h@tachibana-u.ac.jp

IntechOpen

© 2022 The Author(s). Licensee IntechOpen. This chapter is distributed under the terms of the Creative Commons Attribution License (http://creativecommons.org/licenses/by/3.0), which permits unrestricted use, distribution, and reproduction in any medium, provided the original work is properly cited.

References

[1] Beaulieu LD, Schneider C. Effects of repetitive peripheral magnetic stimulation on normal or impaired motor control. A review. Neurophysiologie Clinique. 2013;**43**:251-260. DOI: 10.1016/j.neucli.2013.05.003

[2] Barker AT. An introduction to the basic principles of magnetic nerve stimulation. Journal of Clinical Neurophysiology. 1991;**8**:26-37. DOI: 10.1097/00004691-199101000-00005

[3] Sakai K, Yasufuku Y, Kamo T, Ota E, Momosaki R. Repetitive peripheral magnetic stimulation for impairment and disability in people after stroke. Stroke. 2020;**51**:e105-e106. DOI: 10.1002/14651858.CD011968.pub3

[4] Han TR, Shin HI, Kim IS. Magnetic stimulation of the quadriceps femoris muscle: Comparison of pain with electrical stimulation. American Journal of Physical Medicine & Rehabilitation. 2006;**85**:593-599. DOI: 10.1097/01.phm.0000223239.93539.fe

[5] Nito M, Katagiri N, Yoshida K, Koseki T, Kudo D, Nanba S, et al. Repetitive peripheral magnetic stimulation of wrist extensors enhances cortical excitability and motor performance in healthy individuals. Frontiers in Neuroscience. 2021;**15**:632716. DOI: 10.3389/fnins.2021.632716

[6] Kumru H, Albu S, Rothwell J, Leon D, Flores C, Opisso E, et al. Modulation of motor cortex excitability by paired peripheral and transcranial magnetic stimulation. Clinical Neurophysiology. 2017;**128**:2043-2047. DOI: 10.1016/j.clinph.2017.06.041

[7] Krause P, Straube A. Peripheral repetitive magnetic stimulation induces intracortical inhibition in healthy subjects. Neurological Research. 2008;**30**:690-694. DOI: 10.1179/174313208X297959

[8] Asao A, Ikeda H, Nomura T, Shibuya K. Short-term session of repetitive peripheral magnetic stimulation combined with motor imagery facilitates corticospinal excitability in healthy human participants. Neuroreport. 2019;**30**:562-566. DOI: 10.1097/WNR.0000000000001245

[9] Asao A, Wada K, Nomura T, Shibuya K. Time course changes in corticospinal excitability during repetitive peripheral magnetic stimulation combined with motor imagery. Neuroscience Letters. 2022;**771**:136427. DOI: 10.1016/j.neulet.2021.136427

[10] Yang SS, Jee S, Hwang SL, Sohn MK. Strengthening of quadriceps by neuromuscular magnetic stimulation in healthy subjects. PM & R : The Journal of Injury, Function, and Rehabilitation. 2017;**9**:767-773. DOI: 10.1016/j.pmrj.2016.12.002

[11] Stolting MN, Arnold AS, Haralampieva D, Handschin C, Sulser T, Eberli D. Magnetic stimulation supports muscle and nerve regeneration after trauma in mice. Muscle & Nerve. 2016;**53**:598-607. DOI: 10.1002/mus.24780

[12] Hirono T, Ikezoe T, Taniguchi M, Nojiri S, Tanaka H, Ichihashi N. Acute effects of repetitive peripheral magnetic stimulation following low-intensity isometric exercise on muscle swelling for selective muscle in healthy young men. Electromagnetic Biology and Medicine. 2021;**40**:420-427. DOI: 10.1080/15368378.2021.1907402

[13] Schoenfeld BJ. Potential mechanisms for a role of metabolic stress in hypertrophic adaptations to resistance training. Sports Medicine. 2013;**43**:179-194. DOI: 10.1007/s40279-013-0017-1

[14] Hirono T, Ikezoe T, Taniguchi M, Tanaka H, Saeki J, Yagi M, et al. Relationship between muscle swelling and hypertrophy induced by resistance training. Journal of Strength and Conditioning Research. 2022;**36**:359-364. DOI: 10.1519/JSC.0000000000003478

[15] Baek J, Park N, Lee B, Jee S, Yang S, Kang S. Effects of repetitive peripheral magnetic stimulation over vastus lateralis in patients after hip replacement surgery. Annals of Rehabilitation Medicine. 2018;**42**:67-75. DOI: 10.5535/arm.2018.42.1.67

[16] Yavuzer G, Selles R, Sezer N, Sütbeyaz S, Bussmann JB, Köseoğlu F, et al. Mirror therapy improves hand function in subacute stroke: A randomized controlled trial. Archives of Physical Medicine and Rehabilitation. 2008;**89**:393-398. DOI: 10.1016/j.apmr.2007.08.162

[17] Liu M, Fujiwara T, Shindo K, Kasashima Y, Otaka Y, Tsuji T, et al. Newer challenges to restore hemiparetic upper extremity after stroke: HANDS therapy and BMI neurorehabilitation. Hong Kong Physiotherapy Journal. 2012;**30**:83-92

[18] Jiang YF, Zhang D, Zhang J, Hai H, Zhao YY, Ma YW. A randomized controlled trial of repetitive peripheral magnetic stimulation applied in early subacute stroke: Effects on severe upper-limb impairment. Clinical Rehabilitation. 2022;**36**:693-702. DOI: 10.1177/02692155211072189

[19] Fernandez-Lobera M, Morales M, Valls-Solé J. Repetitive peripheral magnetic stimulation for the assessment of wrist spasticity: Reliability, validation and correlation with clinical measures. Disability and Rehabilitation. 2021:1-11. DOI: 10.1080/09638288.2021.1925979

[20] Arya KN, Pandian S, Bhatnagar N, Sharma A. Rehabilitation of the shoulder subluxation based on ultrasonographic findings among post stroke subjects: A case series. Neurology India. 2021;**69**:1309-1317. DOI: 10.4103/0028-3886.329613

[21] Fujimura K, Kagaya H, Endou C, Ishihara A, Nishigaya K, Muroguchi K, et al. Effects of repetitive peripheral magnetic stimulation on shoulder subluxations caused by stroke: A preliminary study. Neuromodulation. 2020;**23**:847-851. DOI: 10.1111/ner.13064

[22] Krewer C, Hartl S, Müller F, Koenig E. Effects of repetitive peripheral magnetic stimulation on upper-limb spasticity and impairment in patients with spastic hemiparesis: A randomized, double-blind, sham-controlled study. Archives of Physical Medicine and Rehabilitation. 2014;**95**:1039-1047. DOI: 10.1016/j.apmr.2014.02.003

[23] Kinoshita S, Ikeda K, Hama M, Suzuki S, Abo M. Repetitive peripheral magnetic stimulation combined with intensive physical therapy for gait disturbance after hemorrhagic stroke:

An open-label case series. International Journal of Rehabilitation Research. 2020;**43**:235-239. DOI: 10.1097/MRR.0000000000000416

[24] Beaulieu LD, Massé-Alarie H, Brouwer B, Schneider C. Noninvasive neurostimulation in chronic stroke: A double-blind randomized sham-controlled testing of clinical and corticomotor effects. Topics in Stroke Rehabilitation. 2015;**22**:8-17. DOI: 10.1179/1074935714Z.0000000032

Chapter 4

Possibility of Using a VR System as an Action Observation Therapeutical Technique

Jaroslav Langer, Monika Šorfová and David Ravnik

Abstract

In recent years, 3D virtual reality (VR) systems are increasingly finding their way into biomedical applications. Nevertheless, in most cases a 3D VR is being used as an interactive system (such as Xbox Kinect or Playstation VR). These interactive systems, however effective they may have proven, not only limit use of 3D VR in patients incapable to engage in these systems due to their physical or mental disability, but also put significant requirements on medical institutions for an equipment, medical personal, and therefore institutional budget. In this article, we are proposing a 3D VR as an stand-alone action observation training device, which could limit requirements associated with abovementioned interactive systems due to its capability to stimulate a mirror neuron system of human brain, while adding minimal demands on both patient and medical facility. Research studies that confirm activity in the motor cortex will be described. We focus on the literature that describes theories, models, and experimental studies dealing with the effects of motion observations that are involved in the control and final performance of motor skills.

Keywords: virtual reality, mirror neuron, action observation, motor imagery

1. Introduction

3D virtual reality (VR) is currently being used mainly for gaming purposes. However, there is an increasing number of VR implementations in fields of sports training and rehabilitation. The system being used as a VR training system is usually an interactive gaming system (e.g., Playstation VR, Nintendo Wii…). Nevertheless, a simple action observation (AO) using 3D VR system without its interactive component is also an interesting, if not regularly implemented, option to increase a therapy time without an involvement of therapist in the process, due to AO's capability to activate mirror neuron network. In case the use of VR in such a way is possible, it might open up new ways of therapeutical approaches in many patient cases, where there is a lack of cooperation with patient and the interactive VR system would not be applicable.

2. Mirror neuron

A theory of the specific premotor brain cells, which are activated not only during actual motor execution of a movement, but also during observing the movement, was first formulated in 1992 by si Pellegrino [1]. An activation in the F5 area of the makak's brain was found, which was the same for particular movement components (such as a grasp) as for an observation of a human grasping an object. This provided a mechanism for explanation of AO's relation to the motor planning. A consequential research [2] described 532 specific neuron cells in abovementioned cortex area, which were named "mirror neurons" (MNs). Most of the newly found structures were reacting to the movement related to a hand grasp and about 30% of them were involved in specific manipulations and movements. Therefore, the theory about MN being an inherent part of the motor planning was developed.

2.1 A road to human trials

In subsequential studies, other major brain areas containing MN were described. Also different cells were found to have different activation stimulus (e.g., MN activated only during AO, MN activated during AO and motor execution...). However most of the research was still focused on the F5 brain area of monkey's brain, where the highest number of MN was found, mainly due to inaccurate or unsafe observing methods for human trials.

Nowadays (03/2022) PubMed returns over 200 results to search of "mirror neurons AND human". Usually, an activity of MN system is measured by functional MRI. A problem is in contrast agents, which are normally used in the monkey trials (most often monocrystalic iron oxide nanoparticles), but are toxic for the human bodies [3].

For differentiation of specific neuron cells via fMRI is theoretically possible solution in natural neuron adaptation on stimulus-neural response decreases with stimulation. For MN, the decrease should be present both via observing and via executing movement. There are studies available [4] that confirm this theory, whereas others did not find any MN adaptation signs in humans [5] or in monkeys [6].

However, there is an evidence for neuron activity in same regions of premotor cortex during action observation for humans and monkeys [7].

In 2012, Molenberghse et al. described on fMRI (n = 125) 14 areas with the corresponding activity to the stimulus as with the monkey brains. These areas mainly contain prefrontal gyrus, ventral and dorsal motor cortex an parietal lobe during action observation; however, MN characteristic activity was also found in the amygdala, insula, and other regions of cortex during emotional and acoustic stimulation. In total there was described activity corresponding to MNs in 34 Brodmann areas of the human brain. Although the authors conclude the paper with the observation that, taking into account the findings from monkey brains, it is unlikely that all the 34 regions directly contain MN cells, there is found the recurrent response of the human brain to sensory (optical, auditory, and emotional) stimuli, as well as downstream activity in cortical areas, corresponding to the presence of MN [8].

2.2 Stimulation of MN as a way to train motor skills

The abovementioned findings open up, among other things, the possibility of using the MN stimulation as a training or therapeutic tool. Due to the activation of some MN during the execution and monitoring of the movement, and provided that these MN are involved in movement imagery and planning, their targeted involvement can be as a tool for training motor functions. In practice, the targeted MN can be set into two types: the aforementioned action observation and a motor imagery (MI).

3. Action observation and a clinical use

The use of AO in the treatment of motor deficits is a relatively well-documented phenomenon. Some authors refer to AO directly as to a mechanism activating MN that mediates sensory and emotional learning, as well as learning from an observation of movement, and thus represents the potential for the use of AO and its action through MN as a passive rehabilitation and learning technique for both cognitive-behavioral and motor function [9].

The effect of independent AO on postural stability and movement coordination has been described. For example, Son & Kang [10] observed another person performing the same test between two measurements and found a significant increase in stability during Y-balance test compared with the control group. Given that observation of another person performing the test was the only difference in the test protocol between the test and control groups, the authors conclude that AO, even without the use of an additional training technique, has the potential to affect stability.

Similarly, Gatti et al. [11], in their comparison of the AO and balance effect training, focus on the effect of AO on the stability. The authors measured the changes in center of pressure (COP) in stance modifications. The sample of probands (n = 79) was divided into three groups with different training protocols (AO, AO with a movement imitation, balance training) and one control group. The balance training consisted of a series of coordination and stability demanding movements (walking on the balance beam, standing on a trampoline on one leg, standing on a roller, etc.). The video used showed the same movements performed by a professional athlete. According to the results of this work, the AO together with the imitation of the movements even appears to be an equivalent training tool to increase postural control as a stand-alone balance training (effect size ES [0,7]) compared with the control group. AO alone then has a lower effect size (ES [0.3]), but still it is significant.

There has also been described an increase in muscle strength in the hand movement after AO therapy. For example, Porro et al. [12] found that of the 82 participants in the experiments, for the physical training, group muscle strength was 50% higher than baseline values were, but even in the AO-only intervention group, this change was significant (+33%) compared with the baseline values. There was no significant change in the control group.

The findings open the question of using AO for motor stability learning with temporarily immobile patients or in specific motor deficits.

A positive effect of AO intervention for post-stroke patients has also been described. Nevertheless, AO appears to be the most effective as an addition to execution of an observed activity (overall balance index 2.3 ± 2.0 before and 1.2 ± 0.8 post-test; mEFAP 102.2 ± 45.5 pre and 54.2 ± 41.4 post-test) [13].

For children and adolescents with Down syndrome, the use of "therapeutic virtual reality" represents an opportunity to significantly improve coordination and stability of movement and, last but not least, the fun in exercise (46.86 + 7.98 before, 53.57 + 1.99 after therapy in the KTK motor test) [14]. Lohse et al. [15] in a systematic review and meta-analysis of 26 papers describing the effect of VR in the rehabilitation of stroke patients found that using VR therapy results in significant effect compared with conventional therapeutic methods in standard motor tests results (ES [0.48]), as well as in functional tests ("ADL" tests; ES [0.58]). VR games (XBox 360 Kinect) were also used to successfully influence the coordination skills of children with central coordination disorder as measured by the DCDQ test ($p = 0.003$ for $\alpha = 0{,}05$) [16]. And in addition to the aforementioned collection of work dedicated to MN activity on fMRI, there are also five studies measuring EEG from which the result is that both AO and mirror therapies increase the possibility of motor unit inhibition in spasticity [17].

Hebert [18] showed that AO has a positive effect on coordination, the ability to plan and to learn, even for complex activities and movements such as a "speed stacking" (building pyramids from the cups). In three training rounds of VR, the probands in the first round were slower than in the second round (Cohen's $d = 0.64$) and in the second round they were slower than in the third round (Cohen's $d = 0.56$).

LoJacono et al. then showed that training in a virtual environment can change the movement strategy in a real environment. Between two "cross obstacle" tests in the real environment, probands ($n = 40$) underwent training of the same movement on a treadmill with an obstacle projected using VR. It was confirmed that the training effect is already observable in the virtual environment ($F[3,36] = 5.10$, $p = .01$, $\eta 2 = 0.30$), and even that there is a change in movement strategy in the real environment and that the movement after the training is performed more safely ($F[4,34] = 4.42$, $p = .01$, $\eta 2 = .34$) [19].

4. Motor imagery and its clinical use

From the available evidence, MN system activity is present not only at the abovementioned observation, but also when imagining movement [20–23]. At first glance, thus the MI appears to be a substitutable mechanism for AO and VR systems.

However, specific studies dedicated to this possibility seem to suggest otherwise. According to data from Gonzalez-Rosa et al. from EEG imaging during the implementation of complex movements of all four limbs during the training, there is an increase in activity for the both training mechanisms ($F(4, 52) = 4.18$, $p = 0.02$), but with a significantly higher MN activation during AO in both the parietal lobe ($p = 0.03$) and frontal lobe ($p = 0.79$) compared with MI training. Then, during the execution of the trained movement, the observable effect during kinematic analysis in movement speed ($F(5,130) = 6.58$, $p < 0.01$), as well as a group effect [$F(2, 26) = 3.73$, $p = 0.03$] with a significant difference between the AO and MI groups ($p = 0.03$) occurred. The results, among others, were interpreted by the authors as showing lower MN activation and thus lower clinical effect of MI, probably due to the imagery of unspecified movement difficult for probands to imagine specifically. The authors open a discussion on the imaginative abilities of the probands [24].

Similarly, Neuper et al. describe MN activation in MI, but lower than in AO [25]. And Bakker et al. [26], measuring brain excitability, found an effect of imagining a simple dorsiflexion leg movement, but for a complex movement (walking), this effect was only evident for probands with above-average excitability for the simple movement.

Thus, although MI appears to be a suitable alternative to therapies using AO, the resulting activation can be highly variable. In its use, reliance must be placed on the interindividual psychomotor abilities of the patients and during the course of therapy there is no option beyond the relatively complicated EEG measurement or fMRI to check for correct implementation of the therapy. In contrast, in AO, the therapy can act on relatively complex and specific motor functions (grip, dorsiflexion of the leg, etc.) in a specific way, which is easily repeatable in the case of video-assisted AO.

Based on the different brain activity and the different effects of each type of training in the above works, we hypothesize that using AO visual feedback contributes positively to the activation of the MN system and thus potentially leading to a higher training effects. The aforementioned findings pointing to a lower effectiveness of MI training compared with AO, as well as to interindividual differences in the effect of MI on brain activity (especially in more complex movements), represent potential limitations to the use of MI in clinical practice.

5. Mechanisms in AO and MI

Differences between AO and MI are not only in clinical effects but also in mechanisms of their effects on brain activity—AO has a higher proportion of visual feedback, thus providing a concrete representation of the trained movement. Following a different principle of MN activation, different activity of individual brain regions was found.

During AO, activity was observed mainly in the brain regions ventral and dorsal premotor cortex (VPC, DPC), in the upper and inferior parietal lobe, in the sulcus temporalis superior, and in the dorsolateral prefrontal cortex. Combination of these areas is called an "action observation network" (AON). In some of these areas, particularly in the VPC, in the inferior temporal lobe and in the sulcus temporalis superior, the presence of MN has been described [27]. AON activity is also associated with an increase in motor-evoked potentials, i.e., with an increase in corticospinal excitability.

During MI, activity is observable in the supplementary motor area, in the primary motor area, the premotor area, the basal ganglia area, and the cerebellum, areas similar to those involved in real movement; however, the activity in these areas is in comparison to the actual execution of the movement different—in MI, the activity of the premotor cortex in particular is significantly lower [28]. At the same time, the activated regions differ according to the type of motor imagery. For example, the parietal lobe is activated similarly in both kinesthetic and visual imagery, but there are observable variations in motor and visual centers [29–30]. It is therefore necessary to differentiate and correctly instruct the different modalities of MI depending on the intended activation.

6. VR parameters to optimize results

With the assumption that VR can be an effective tool to influence MN and thus motor function, the question arises on what parameters the VR used should meet.

Perez-Marcos [31] talks in his overview of VR technology about four qualities of VR environments: immersion, interaction, sensorimotor capabilities, and illusion. Immersion is fundamental potential advantage of 3D VR systems. However, it is not just about the type of projection, but about the overall way in which the virtual environment is mediated. Immersivity can also be supported by other sensory perceptions (e.g., audio, tactile...).

Above all, the possibility of interaction increases the fidelity of the experience. Nevertheless it seems that the immersiveness induced by the use of appropriate inputs can, over time, "burn out" if there is no opportunity to interact with the virtual environment. The simplest form of the interaction is said to be the response of the image to the movement of the head—by looking around in the virtual environment. Notwithstanding it can be extended to include for example image response to an observer activity or, in the case of robotic systems, mechanisms using biofeedback.

Sensorimotor interactions allow for another "layer" of interaction with the virtual environment. One of the top forms is the mentioned biofeedback (e.g., EMG-driven exoskeleton), or the mediation of specific tactile sensations related to our activity in the projected image. In practical applications, it is usually a vibrating game system controller. More advanced sensorimotor response can be provided by some robotic systems.

In the context of VR, illusion is the last "stage" in the quality of the environment, including all the previous ones. An ideal VR system would be able to provide such a high immersiveness, such a high level of interaction and such faithful sensorimotor information, that it would be possible to fully feel and fully "trust" in one's presence in a virtual environment.

Wenk et al. elaborated, in their comparison of the different VR principles, the difference between immersive (3D) virtual reality (IVR) and 2D VR (screen) as to an impact on the movement quality as assessed by the motor and cognitive tests. The study participants placed objects on the marks in the virtual environment while counting them. During the test, task duration, straightness of trajectory of movement, speed of movement, and cognitive load were measured. In the IVR environment, compared with the 2D VR, the tests were performed faster (ES [0.7519]) and with a more direct trajectory (ES [0.7194]) [32]. And Panek et al. described lower brain activity during 2D VR observation compared with observing therapist performing the movement. These findings seem to suggest that the higher the immersion, the higher the activity [33].

7. Suggestion of VR for motor training via AO

As a consequence of the abovementioned findings, we argue it is possible to suggest principles for VR implementation to the clinical practice. First of all, the chosen system should provide the highest possible level of immersion possible. The use of 3D VR systems over 2D VR is therefore preferable. The video chosen for the intervention should be made in such a way that the 3D environment presented provides the most "real life experience" possible - "first person" video format is preferable over third-person game animations. The movements chosen for the AO should be presented specifically and simply enough so that observers can relate to their execution—e.g., grabbing a ball in the video is preferable over the video of painting a picture on canvas.

With abovementioned principles, it is theoretically possible to start using VR as stand-alone system for AO, without the use of interactive system. Although the implementation of interactive component is arguably beneficial (at least to the brain activity), the use of VR for AO poses possibility to intervene in patient cases, where an active cooperation is (for whatever reason) not possible.

8. Conclusion

In this article, we aimed to summarize the principles involved in action observation via VR system used as a stand-alone action observation training device. Although the published studies indicate that in many cases (e.g., balance tests, coordination skills, etc.) the implementation of interactive component is arguably beneficial (at least to the brain activity), the use of VR for AO poses possibility to intervene in patient cases, where an active cooperation is (for whatever reason) not possible. With the information gained from our literature research, we are suggesting the parameters for VR video suitable for AO training. Although more research and thorough clinical trials for this principle are definitely needed, the use of 3D VR without interactive component involved seems to pose an interesting opportunity for implementing relatively new and attractive technology to increase efficiency of standard therapeutical approaches.

Acknowledgements

Written as part of project: SVV 260599 2020 -2022, PROGRES, Cooperation 2022 - 2026.

Conflict of interest

The authors declare no conflict of interest.

Author details

Jaroslav Langer[1*], Monika Šorfová[1] and David Ravnik[2]

1 UK FTVS, Prague, Czechia

2 Faculty of Health Sciences, University of Primorska, Slovenia

*Address all correspondence to: jarosl.langer@gmail.com

IntechOpen

© 2022 The Author(s). Licensee IntechOpen. This chapter is distributed under the terms of the Creative Commons Attribution License (http://creativecommons.org/licenses/by/3.0), which permits unrestricted use, distribution, and reproduction in any medium, provided the original work is properly cited.

References

[1] di Pellegrino G, Fadiga L, Fogassi L, Gallese V, Rizzolatti G. Understanding motor events: A neurophysiological study. Experimental Brain Research. 1992;**91**(1):176-180. DOI: 10.1007/BF00230027

[2] Gallese V, Fadiga L, Fogassi L, Rizzolatti G. Action recognition in the premotor cortex. Brain: A. Journal of Neurology. 1996;**119**(Pt 2):593-609. DOI: 10.1093/brain/119.2.593

[3] Kilner JM, Lemon RN. What we know currently about Mirror neurons. Current Biology. 2013;**23**(23):R1057-R1062. DOI: 10.1016/j.cub.2013.10.051

[4] Kilner JM, Neal A, Weiskopf N, Friston KJ, Frith CD. Evidence of Mirror neurons in human inferior frontal gyrus. Journal of Neuroscience. 2009;**29**(32):10153-10159. DOI: 10.1523/JNEUROSCI.2668-09.2009

[5] Lingnau A, Gesierich B, Caramazza A. Asymmetric fMRI adaptation reveals no evidence for mirror neurons in humans. Proceedings of the National Academy of Sciences. 2009;**106**(24):9925-9930. DOI: 10.1073/pnas.0902262106

[6] Caggiano V, Pomper JK, Fleischer F, Fogassi L, Giese M, Thier P. Mirror neurons in monkey area F5 do not adapt to the observation of repeated actions. Nature Communications. 2013;**4**(1):1433. DOI: 10.1038/ncomms2419

[7] Buccino G, Binkofski F, Riggio L. The mirror neuron system and action recognition. Brain and Language. 2004;**89**(2):370-376. DOI: 10.1016/S0093-934X(03)00356-0

[8] Molenberghs P, Cunnington R, Mattingley JB. Brain regions with mirror properties: A meta-analysis of 125 human fMRI studies. Neuroscience & Biobehavioral Reviews. 2012;**36**(1):341-349. DOI: 10.1016/j.neubiorev.2011.07.004

[9] Mathon B. Les neurones miroirs: De l'anatomie aux implications physiopathologiques et thérapeutiques. Revue Neurologique. 2013;**169**(4):285-290. DOI: 10.1016/j.neurol.2012.10.008

[10] Son SM, Kang KW. Effect of action observation training using Y-balance on balance capability in young adults. The Journal of Korean Physical Therapy. 2020;**32**(2):65-69. DOI: 10.18857/jkpt.2020.32.2.65

[11] Gatti R, Sarasso E, Pelachin M, Agosta F, Filippi M, Tettamanti A. Can action observation modulate balance performance in healthy subjects? Archives of Physiotherapy. 2019;**9**(1):1. DOI: 10.1186/s40945-018-0053-0

[12] Porro CA, Facchin P, Fusi S, Dri G, Fadiga L. Enhancement of force after action observation. Neuropsychologia. 2007;**45**(13):3114-3121. DOI: 10.1016/j.neuropsychologia.2007.06.016

[13] Lee HJ, Kim YM, Lee DK. The effects of action observation training and mirror therapy on gait and balance in stroke patients. Journal of Physical Therapy Science. 2017;**29**(3):523-526. DOI: 10.1589/jpts.29.523

[14] Gouveia Reis JR, Merussi Neiva C, Pessoa Filho DM, Gomes Ciolac E, Lopes Verardi CE, da Cruz Siqueira LO, et al. Virtual reality therapy: Motor coordination and balance analysis in children and teenagers with down syndrome. /Terapia De Realidad virtual: Coordinacionmotora Y Analisis Del Equilibrio En Niñosy

Adolescentes con Sindrome De Down. Motricidad: European Journal of Human Movement. 2017;**38**:53-67

[15] Lohse KR, Hilderman CGE, Cheung KL, Tatla S, Loos HFMV d. Virtual reality therapy for adults post-stroke: A systematic review and Meta-analysis exploring virtual environments and commercial games in therapy. PLoS One. 2014;**9**(3):e93318. DOI: 10.1371/journal.pone.0093318

[16] Trivedi DG, Dwivedi AK, Tripathi HJ, Varma TV, Bharmbhatt HB, Prabhakar KB. To study the effectiveness of virtual reality on coordination of children with developmental coordination disorder: A pilot study. International Journal of Recent Scientific Research. 2021;**12**(07):42272-42275. DOI: 10.24327/ijrsr.2021.1207.6061

[17] Zhang JJQ, Fong KNK, Welage N, Liu KPY. The activation of the Mirror neuron system during action observation and action execution with Mirror visual feedback in stroke: A systematic review. Neural Plasticity. 2018;**2018**:1-14. DOI: 10.1155/2018/2321045

[18] Hebert E. The effects of observing a learning model (or two) on motor skill acquisition. Journal of Motor Learning & Development. 2018;**6**(1):4-17

[19] LoJacono CT, MacPherson RP, Kuznetsov NA, Raisbeck LD, Ross SE, Rhea CK. Obstacle crossing in a virtual environment transfers to a real environment. Journal of Motor Learning & Development. 2018;**6**(2):234-249

[20] Cattaneo L, Rizzolatti G. The mirror neuron system. Archives of Neurology. 2009;**66**(5):557-560. DOI: 10.1001/archneurol.2009.41

[21] Johnson S. Selective activation of a Parietofrontal circuit during implicitly imagined Prehension. NeuroImage. 2002;**17**(4):1693-1704. DOI: 10.1006/nimg.2002.1265

[22] Lotze M, Montoya P, Erb M, Hülsmann E, Flor H, Klose U, et al. Activation of cortical and cerebellar motor areas during executed and imagined hand movements: An fMRI study. Journal of Cognitive Neuroscience. 1999;**11**(5):491-501. DOI: 10.1162/089892999563553

[23] Wang L, Zhang J, Zhang Y, Yan R, Liu H, Qiu M. Conditional granger causality analysis of effective connectivity during motor imagery and motor execution in stroke patients. BioMed Research International. 2016;**2016**:1-9. DOI: 10.1155/2016/3870863

[24] Gonzalez-Rosa JJ, Natali F, Tettamanti A, Cursi M, Velikova S, Comi G, et al. Action observation and motor imagery in performance of complex movements: Evidence from EEG and kinematics analysis. Behavioural Brain Research. 2015;**281**:290-300. DOI: 10.1016/j.bbr.2014.12.016

[25] Neuper C, Scherer R, Reiner M, Pfurtscheller G. Imagery of motor actions: Differential effects of kinesthetic and visual–motor mode of imagery in single-trial EEG. Cognitive Brain Research. 2005;**25**(3):668-677. DOI: 10.1016/j.cogbrainres.2005.08.014

[26] Bakker M, Overeem S, Snijders AH, Borm G, van Elswijk G, Toni I, et al. Motor imagery of foot dorsiflexion and gait: Effects on corticospinal excitability. Clinical Neurophysiology. 2008;**119**(11):2519-2527. DOI: 10.1016/j.clinph.2008.07.282

[27] Rizzolatti G, Craighero L. THE MIRROR-NEURON SYSTEM. Annual Review of Neuroscience.

2004;**27**(1):169-192. DOI: 10.1146/annurev.neuro.27.070203.144230

[28] Hétu S, Grégoire M, Saimpont A, Coll M-P, Eugène F, Michon P-E, et al. The neural network of motor imagery: An ALE meta-analysis. Neuroscience & Biobehavioral Reviews. 2013;**37**(5): 930-949. DOI: 10.1016/j.neubiorev.2013.03.017

[29] Guillot A, Collet C, Nguyen VA, Malouin F, Richards C, Doyon J. Brain activity during visual versus kinesthetic imagery: An fMRI study. Human Brain Mapping. 2009;**30**(7):2157-2172. DOI: 10.1002/hbm.20658

[30] Mizuguchi N, Nakata H, Uchida Y, Kanosue K. Motor imagery and sport performance. The Journal of Physical Fitness and Sports Medicine. 2012;**1**(1):103-111. DOI: 10.7600/jpfsm.1.103

[31] Perez-Marcos D. Virtual reality experiences, embodiment, videogames and their dimensions in neurorehabilitation. Journal of Neuroengineering and Rehabilitation. 2018;**15**(1):113. DOI: 10.1186/s12984-018-0461-0

[32] Wenk N, Penalver-Andres J, Palma R, Buetler KA, Muri R, Nef T, et al. Reaching in several realities: Motor and cognitive benefits of different visualization technologies. In: 2019 IEEE 16th International Conference on Rehabilitation Robotics (ICORR). Toronto, ON, Canada: IEEE; 2019. pp. 1037-1042. DOI: 10.1109/ICORR.2019.8779366

[33] Pánek D, Nováková T, Brunovský M, Košťálová J, Pavlů D. The effect of active movement and passive monitoring of the same movement on electric brain activity. Rehabilitace a fyzikální lékařství. 2018;**2018**(25):152-157

Section 2

Clinical Research

Chapter 5

Effect of Unilateral Neglect with Basal Ganglia Bleed in Stroke Survivor

Ashna Sinha and Meena Gupta

Abstract

Basal ganglia accounts to most common site of hemorrhagic stroke (50%). Right hemisphere lesions that are restricted to basal ganglia are responsible for perceptual disorders such as unilateral neglect. Unilateral Neglect is a very common perceptual disorder that occurs after stroke. Unilateral neglect when compared to the stroke severity results in poor overall recovery. It may involve longer hospitalization period, functional dependency, long term disability in ADLs as well as increased risk of falls. Postural imbalance is more prevalent with right hemisphere lesions. Stroke survivors with right hemisphere damage have less ability to ambulate. As the stroke patient's balance is impaired and can lead to serious consequences like falls. So, if we know the questions related to balance and gait in stroke patients then it would be very important for us to understand these two physical capabilities among the hemiparetic subjects. It is therefore believed that it will lead to a better direction regarding the rehabilitation of these stroke patients. The case report presented here describes the clinical presentation of a right basal ganglia bleed patient who had unilateral neglect.

Keywords: unilateral neglect, BG bleed, Catherine Bergego scale, Fugl Meyer assessment

1. Introduction

Stroke is the 3rd major cause of morbidity and mortality in many countries. It is basically of three types: ischemic, thrombotic & hemorrhagic. Ischemic stroke results from reduced blood supply, thrombotic stroke results from clot formation in a blood vessel whereas hemorrhagic stroke results from rupture of blood vessel. The latter is of following two types: intracerebral and subarachnoid [1]. Among the intracerebral hemorrhage, basal ganglia bleed is most common. It usually results from poorly controlled or long-standing hypertension [2]. Cigarette smoking and alcohol consumption further adds on to the risk of developing such stroke. Basal ganglia accounts to most common site of hemorrhagic stroke (50%). Other sites are cerebral lobes (10%), pons & brainstem (10–20%), thalamus (15%) and cerebellum (10%) [2, 3]. Right side cortical stroke is closely related to perceptual disorders. Many studies suggests that right hemisphere lesions that are restricted to

IntechOpen

basal ganglia are responsible for perceptual disorders such as unilateral neglect [4]. Unilateral Neglect is a very common perceptual disorder that occurs after stroke. It can be defined as the inability to respond, report or orient to stimuli on contralateral side to brain lesion [5]. ULN is of different types. On the basis of behavior that is elicited it is classified into sensory, motor, and representational type and on the basis of abnormal behavior distribution ULN is of personal & spatial type [6]. Unilateral neglect can be assessed by many qualitative as well as quantitative tools such as Behavioral Inattention Test, Cancelation test, Line bisection test, Copying & drawing test, Catherine Bergego Scale etc. Unilateral neglect when compared to the stroke severity results in poor overall recovery. It may involve longer hospitalization period, functional dependency, long term disability in ADLs as well as increased risk of falls [7]. Postural imbalance is more prevalent with right hemisphere lesions. Stroke survivors with right hemisphere damage have less ability to ambulate. This is because they have lesser ability to shift weight on the non-paretic leg [8]. Acquiring independence of gait is one of the prime goals in rehabilitation of stroke subjects. Unilateral Neglect leads to poor gait recovery of activity of daily living as well as gait [9, 10]. Unilateral neglect when clubbed with cognitive impairment has a negative impact on independent gait recovery. Thus, this indicates that the unilateral neglect when combined with cognitive impairments is a strong negative predictor for independent gait [11]. Postural instability is the main cause of falls & limited functional independence among the stroke patients. Posture deficits as well as balance deficits is very common. This is because the good limb has to bear a greater proportion of the body weight. The correlations of parameters of balance and gait is utmost important for thorough assessment of stroke subjects as well as for their proper rehabilitation. This is because a reliable correlation means that resources used to improve balance could also influence gait. As the stroke patient's balance is impaired and can lead to serious consequences like falls. So, if we know the questions related to balance and gait in stroke patients then it would be very important for us to understand these two physical capabilities among the hemiparetic subjects. It is therefore believed that it will lead to a better direction regarding the rehabilitation of these stroke patients. The case report presented here describes the clinical presentation of a right basal ganglia bleed patient who had unilateral neglect.

2. Case presentation

A 40-year male presented with weakness in left arm & and leg along with difficulties in doing ADLs as well as walking since last 2 years. He also complained of occasional headaches. It is a known Follow up case of right basal ganglia bleed with Left Complete Hemiplegia. 2 years prior to episode of stroke, the patient had gone to pick up his elder son from school. He suddenly felt weakness on left side of his body while he was talking to some other parent on the street. He lost control of his body and fell on the ground. He was then immediately taken to Safdarjung hospital where CT Scan of brain was done which revealed intracranial bleed. His family members then took LAMA from there and admitted the patient to Max Super-Speciality Hospital for further management. NCCT head was done which showed a large hematoma in right basal ganglia region with intraventricular extension and midline shift to the left. The doctors then performed right sided decompressive craniectomy with evacuation of hematoma on 1st Feb 2019. He was managed in ICU on ventilator & necessary support. His condition gradually improved and he was then discharged from the hospital. He received regular physiotherapy sessions during his stay in the hospital. He was advised for cranioplasty after 1 month. He was then admitted in Vimhans hospital on 19th July 2019 for cranioplasty. He underwent regular physiotherapy sessions again during his stay at the hospital. After being discharged from the hospital he did exercises at home but since there was not much improvement even after 2 years so his neurologist referred him for regular PT sessions at hospital's Physiotherapy OPD. Patient has history of hypertension since last 5 years and the medicines he was currently taking for that included Tab levesam 500 mg BD, tab Serta 25 mg OD, tab tryptomer 10 mg BD, tab Napra D 250 mg BD and Pantocid 40 mg OD and anti-hypertensive drugs. Patient has habit cigarette smoking (2–3 cigarettes/week). He lives with his wife and 4 kids who help the patient with his activity of daily living. He lives on first floor of the building which has no lift facility. The staircase has proper railings. So, the patient moves up & down through stairs with support of his family members.

On observation the patient was found to be ectomorphic with left side facial asymmetry. He was wearing a shoulder sling. He had circumductory gait but was using quadripod cane for ambulation. On examination he was alert, attentive & oriented with intact short term & long-term memory but impaired immediate memory. He had slurred speech. He was depressed and had MMSE score 20/30 along-with presence of unilateral neglect. All the cranial nerves were intact except left facial nerve. He had left facial nerve palsy with jaw deviated towards right side. Superficial and deep sensations were impaired. Babinski sign was positive on left side. All the DTRs had grade 3+ except supinator jerk which was normal. Tone was remarkedly increased in left upper & lower limb. PROM was within normal ROM but patient had no AROM. Voluntary Control grading for synergy pattern had grade 0 initially with brunnstorm stage 3. Tremors were present in left hand whenever patient did any activity with concentration. Limb girth for both upper & lower limb was remarkedly reduced. Posture assessment in anterior view revealed lt. shoulder drop, rt. side torso shift, lt side pelvic shift, lt hip hike, foot planterflexion & inversion whereas posture assessment in lateral view showed forward head, posterior pelvic tilt and knee hyperextension.

Balance Assessment was done according to Functional Balance Grade: sitting balance (static & dynamic) had grade 2 score and standing balance (static & dynamic) had grade 1 & 0 respectively. Other outcomes measures used were Modified Rankin Scale (Grade 4), Catherine Bergego Scale (Score 17/30), Fugl Meyer Assessment Scale for stroke (UL = 38, LL = 52; total = 90/226). NCCT Head revealed evidence of gliosis noted in right basal ganglia, adjacent fronto-temporo-parietal region with resulting ex-vacuo changes. Mild herniation of brain parenchyma noted at the site of craniectomy defect. Small gliotic focus noted in left basal ganglia region. (20/07/21). Physiotherapy goals were established for the rehabilitation protocol which continued for the duration of 6 weeks (4 times/week). After completion of the rehabilitation, the outcome measures were re-assessed and the prognosis of the patient was reported (**Tables 1** and **2**).

3. Results

The pre and post assessment score of CBS and FMA have been shown in **Table 3**. After the treatment protocol followed, there was marked improvement in unilateral neglect and sensory-motor recovery following stroke. Overall percentage improvement

PT Goals	
Short term goals	**Long term goals**
• Reduce muscle tone to score 1 (acc. to MAS) • Left extremity VC for synergy pattern will improve by at least grade (0/6 advances to 2/6) through all joints within 6 weeks. • Hold a proper posture (trunk control) for at least one full treatment session with no more than 5 cues within 6 weeks. • Achieve good sitting balance on the Functional Balance Grade • Independently perform all transfers (logrolling, supine to sit, sit to stand, stand to sit) for at least 5 repetitions within 6 weeks. • Improve unilateral neglect with score difference of 10 within 6 weeks. • Independently ambulate for at least 10 minutes on even/uneven terrain with his quad cane within 6 weeks	• Improve fine motor skills • Left extremity VC for synergy pattern will improve to at least a grade 3 through all joints within 12 weeks. • Independently perform all transfers (logrolling, supine to sit, sit to stand, stand to sit) for at least 10 repetitions within 12 weeks. • Hold a proper posture (trunk control) for at least one full treatment session with no cueing within 12 weeks. • Independently ambulate for 20 minutes on even/uneven terrain with his quad cane within 12 weeks. • Promote functional independence with a finalized home exercise program for long- term carryover within 12 weeks.

Table 1.
Physiotherapy goals for intervention.

Week 1	• PROM Lt UL & LL (5 reps) • Rocking movement in sitting position (antero-posterior & medio-lateral 5 reps) • Bridging exercise with support (5 reps) • Table polishing exercises (5 reps) • Table top exercises (5 reps) • Compensatory strategies to work on unilateral neglect • MRP approach: getting up from supine position from affected side
Week 2	• PROM Lt UL & LL (10 reps) • Rocking movement in sitting position (antero-posterior & medio-lateral 10 reps) • Bridging exercise with support (10 reps) • Table polishing exercises (7 reps) and Table top exercises (7 reps) • Compensatory strategies to work on unilateral neglect • MRP approach: sitting up from supine position from unaffected side
Week 3	• Single leg bridging exercise with unaffected leg (5 reps) • Table polishing exercises (10 reps) • Table top exercises (10 reps) • Compensatory strategies to work on unilateral neglect • Stretching of wrist flexors, finger flexors and plantarflexors (3 reps, 10s hold) • Ball kicking with support unaffected limb (5 reps) • MRP approach: • Balanced sitting with reaching activities from upper limb (10 reps) • Sit to stand (5 reps) • Functional Electrical Stimulation: for shoulder elevators (Frequency- 40 Hz, Pulse width- 700 ms and Intensity- 3 mA in channel 1, duration-15 min)

Week 4	• Weight bearing exercise in modified plantigrade position. (5 reps) • Single leg bridging exercise with unaffected leg (10 reps) • Table polishing exercises (12 reps) • Table top exercises (12 reps) • Compensatory strategies to work on unilateral neglect • Stretching of wrist flexors, finger flexors and plantarflexors (5 reps, 15 s hold) • Ball kicking with support of unaffected limb (10 reps) • Obstacle crossing (5 reps) • MRP approach: Sit to stand (10 reps) • Stimulate correct standing alignment (by stimulating hip extension, maintaining knee extension and stimulating ankle dorsiflexors) – 5 reps • Functional Electrical Stimulation: for shoulder elevators & wrist extensors (Frequency- 40 Hz, Pulse width- 700 ms and Intensity- 3 mA in channel 1, duration-15 min)
Week 5	• Bridging exercise with affected leg (5 reps) • Peg board activities • Ball kicking with affected limb (5 reps) • Obstacle crossing (7 reps) • Weight bearing exercise in modified plantigrade position. (7 reps) • Single leg standing with support (5 reps) • MRP approach: To prepare for stance phase (stimulate hip extension, train knee control, train for lateral horizontal pelvic shift) – 5 reps • Functional Electrical Stimulation: for shoulder elevators and wrist extensors (Frequency- 40 Hz, Pulse width- 700 ms and Intensity- 3 mA in channel 1 & 4 mA in channel 2, Mode- Alternate and FES rise SNS- 100 ms & FES extension period- 20 ms)
Week 6	• **Week 6** • Bridging exercise with affected leg (10 reps) • Peg board activities • Ball kicking with affected limb (10 reps) • Obstacle crossing (10 reps) • Weight bearing exercise in modified plantigrade position (10 reps) • Single leg standing with support (10 reps) • MRP approach: To prepare for swing phase (train knee flexion, to stimulate knee extension and foot dorsiflexion at heel strike) – 5 reps • Functional Electrical Stimulation: for shoulder elevators and wrist extensors (Frequency- 40 Hz, Pulse width- 700 ms and Intensity- 3 mA in channel 1 & 4 mA in channel 2, Mode- Alternate and FES rise SNS- 100 ms & FES extension period- 20 ms and duration-15 min)

Table 2.
Intervention protocol.

in FMA score was more for lower extremity (24.44%) than that for upper extremity (11.11%). Percentage improvement for overall FMA score was 14.6%. There was remarkedly more improvement in unilateral neglect (30%) (**Figures 1–3**). There was even significant improvement seen in voluntary control grading for synergy pattern, brunnstorm stages, functional balance grade and modified rankin scale as mentioned in **Table 4**.

Outcome Measures	Pre	Post	Percentage Improvement
Catherine Bergego Scale	17/30	8/30	30%
FMA	UL–38 LL–52 Total–90/226	UL–52(126) LL–74(90) Total–123/226	11.11% 24.44% 14.6%

Table 3.
Pre & post score of CBS and FMA along with percentage improvement.

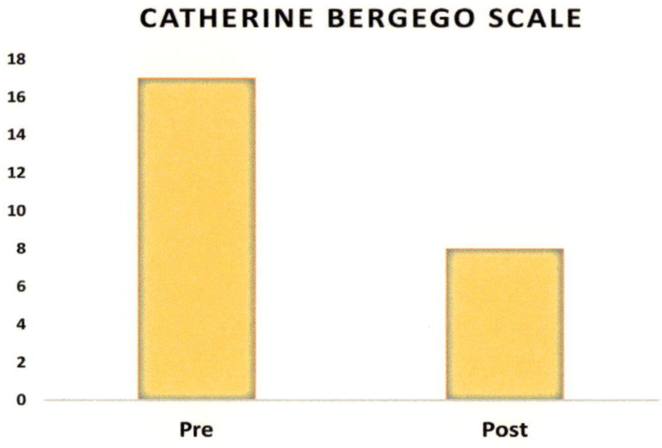

Figure 1.
Pre & post score of CBS (percentage improvement 30%).

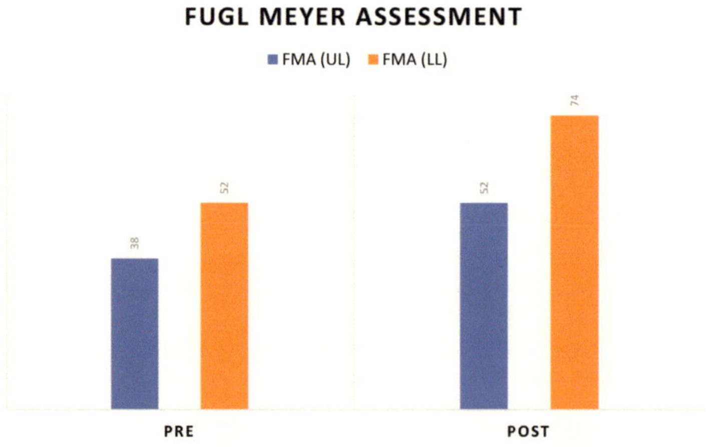

Figure 2.
Pre & post score of FMA for UL & LL (percentage improvement 11.1% & 24.44% respectively).

4. Discussion

The purpose of this study was to find out the effect of unilateral neglect with basal ganglia bleed in stroke survivors. In this study, a stroke survivor with right BG bleed was administered to a six-week intervention protocol following the episode of stroke that occurred 2 years ago. A complete neurological assessment was carried out including

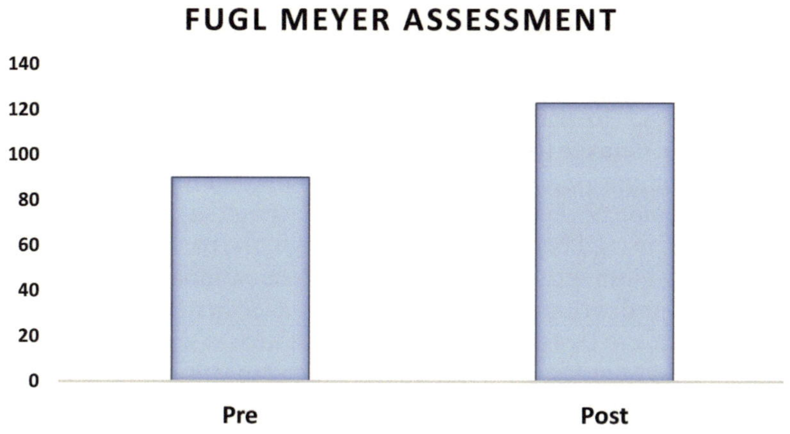

Figure 3.
Pre & post score of FMA (percentage improvement 14.6%).

Outcome Measures	Components	Pre	Post
Voluntary Control Grading for Synergy pattern (Extension Synergy)	UL LL	Grade 0 Grade 0	Grade 1 Grade 2
Brunnstorm stages of stroke recovery		Stage 3	Stage 4
Functional Balance Grade	Sitting • Static • Dynamic Standing • Static • Dynamic	2 2 1 0	3 3 2 1
Modified Rankin Scale		Grade 4	Grade 3
Catherine Bergego Scale		17/30	8/30
FMA	UL LL Total	38 52 90/226	49 74 123/226

Table 4.
Prognosis chart.

certain outcome measures such as MMSE, Voluntary control grading for synergy pattern, Brunnstorm stages of stroke recovery, Functional balance grading, Modified rankin scale, Catherine begego scale and Fugl meyr assessment of sensory & motion functions.

Unilateral Neglect is a very common perceptual disorder that occurs after stroke. It can be defined as the inability to respond, report or orient to stimuli on contralateral side to brain lesion [5]. It is the inability to understand and integrate stimulus and perception from side of body (body neglect) & environment (spatial neglect) [12]. Left sided unilateral neglect which occurs following the episode of right cerebral stroke is more common than the right sided unilateral neglect which occurs following the episode of left cerebral stroke [13]. The prevalence rate of unilateral neglect is 12–100% in case of right hemisphere stroke whereas in case of left hemisphere stroke the prevalence rate ranges between 0 and 76% [14].

Unilateral neglect is more common in acute as well as sub-acute phase. Left hemisphere stroke causes more severe unilateral neglect as compared right hemisphere stroke [15]. Unilateral neglect is mainly caused by right hemisphere damage resulting from stroke which leads to difficulties in attending to stimuli in the left perceptual hemifield. The brain damage that leads to neglect usually involves infarcts in the inferior parietal lobe, temporo-parietal junction & the superior temporal lobe. Unilateral neglect is most common & severe and it occurs following the episode of right cerebral hemisphere infarct [16]. ULN is of different types. On the basis of behavior that is elicited it is classified into sensory, motor, and representational type and on the basis of abnormal behavior distribution ULN is of personal & spatial type [6].

Unilateral neglect can be assessed by many qualitative as well as quantitative tools such as Behavioral Inattention Test, Cancelation test, Line bisection test, Copying & drawing test, Catherine Bergego Scale etc. [6] Out of these tests, in this study CBS has been used to assess the presence as well as the severity of unilateral neglect in stroke subjects. CBS tool has a high sensitivity in evaluating hemi-neglect, and its inter-researcher reliability was highly reliable as r = 0.93 [17]. Unilateral neglect when compared to the stroke severity results in poor overall recovery. It may involve longer hospitalization period, functional dependency, long term disability in ADLs as well as increased risk of falls [18].

Basal ganglia bleed is most common among all types of intracerebral hemorrhages. Long-standing hypertension is one of the major cause responsible for BG bleed. Cigarette smoking and alcohol consumption further adds on to the risk of developing this stroke. Basal ganglia accounts to most common site of hemorrhagic stroke (50%) [2]. Due to the uncommon nature of BG bleed, stroke cases having lesions confined to globus pallidus, caudate & putamen, only limited number of cases have been reported [19]. Neuropsychological problems such as depression occurs very commonly when there are large lesions in basal ganglia [20].

Balance related issues are most commonly seen in stroke survivors. Issues related to balance are often associated risk of falls and mobility problems. Maintenance of balance involves complex interaction of musculoskeletal and neural systems. Out of these, neural components involve motor system, sensory system and higher level cognitive & perceptual processes. Perception and cognition play a very important role in balance control [8]. Postural imbalance is more prevalent with right hemisphere lesions. Stroke survivors with right hemisphere damage have less ability to ambulate. This is because they have lesser ability to shift weight on the non-paretic leg [8]. Perceptual deficit is one of the contributing factors to balance issues which is more commonly seen in right hemisphere stroke lesions. Inappropriate body perception affects the alignment of the body [8].

Acquiring independence of gait is one of the prime goals in rehabilitation of stroke subjects. Unilateral Neglect leads to poor gait recovery of activity of daily living as well as gait [9, 10]. Unilateral neglect when clubbed with cognitive impairment has a negative impact on independent gait recovery. Thus, this indicates that the unilateral neglect when combined with cognitive impairments is a strong negative predictor for independent gait [11].

Postural instability is the main cause of falls & limited functional independence among the stroke patients. Posture deficits as well as balance deficits is very common. This is because the good limb has to bear a greater proportion of the body weight. The correlations of parameters of balance and gait is utmost important for thorough assessment of stroke subjects as well as for their proper rehabilitation. This is because a reliable correlation means that resources used to improve balance could also influence gait. As the stroke patient's balance is impaired and can lead to serious consequences like falls. So, if we know the questions related to balance and gait in stroke patients then it would be very important for us to understand these two physical capabilities among the hemiparetic subjects. It is therefore believed that it will lead to a better direction regarding the rehabilitation of these stroke patients.

Basal ganglia bleed patients are prone to have cognitive impairments [19]. According to a study done by Hochstenbach et al. [21], it is stated that striatum of brain receives inputs from mostly all the cortical regions, thalamus, and limbic system thus playing an integrative role in processing the cognitive information processing. Thus, impairment in cognitive domains occurs following BG patients. Such deficits in BG may lead to deficits in other domain. Aphasia and dysarthria type of speech disorders have a prevalence of about 13% of 240 BG bleed cases. This also occurs due to large lesions in basal ganglia. Damasio et al. 1998 explained about speech disorder having reduced fluency in addition to mild defects of repetition, comprehension & dysarthria [20].

Unilateral neglect is also associated with basal ganglia disorders. Visuospatial functions or hemineglect helps to discriminate between stroke patients and healthy subjects [19]. From a global point of view, destruction of the cortex-striata circuits involving the temporal & parietal lobe leads to difficulties with hemispatial analysis, visual organization and even organization of behavior. Damage of striata impairs performance of striata with respect to spatial cues [22]. According to Harris et al., BG bleed patients have problems of mental rotation of the objects into spatial framework thereby leading to problem of perceptual disorders such as unilateral neglect [23]. Coughlan 1979 explained that with regard to lesion laterality, right BG bleed patients have poorer performance in visuospatial domain whereas left BG bleed patients have more problem in language domain [24]. Thus, rehabilitation of BG bleed patients should always include interventional strategies to work cognitive impairments, unilateral neglect in addition to the basic stroke rehabilitation.

5. Conclusion

This study sheds light upon the effect of unilateral neglect with basal ganglia bleed in stroke survivors. According to the study conducted it was found that perceptual disorders are predominant in right hemisphere lesions. Unilateral neglect being common among the perceptual disorders. Cognitive impairments following the episode of stroke is closely related to such condition depending upon the size of lesion. Neuropsychological dysfunctions such as depression and speech abnormalities such as dysarthria & aphasia are also commonly seen in BG bleed cases. Thus, planning a rehabilitation protocol for such patients should include interventions to work upon unilateral neglect, neuropsychological dysfunctions and speech disorders in addition to improvement in sensory & motor functions for early recovery of stroke survivors. The patient in this study underwent 6 weeks rehabilitation program in the OPD. He was referred to neuro-psychiatrist for medications & counseling for his neuropsychological problems. Referral was also made to speech therapist for his speech problems. He regularly performed home exercise program which was designed by the physical therapist under the supervision of his caregivers. Thus, after following the six-week intervention protocol the patient responded well in terms of sensory-motor recovery and as well showed significant improvement in unilateral neglect.

Author details

Ashna Sinha and Meena Gupta*
Amity Institute of Physiotherapy, Amity University, Noida, Uttar Pradesh, India

*Address all correspondence to: mgupta9@amity.edu

IntechOpen

© 2022 The Author(s). Licensee IntechOpen. This chapter is distributed under the terms of the Creative Commons Attribution License (http://creativecommons.org/licenses/by/3.0), which permits unrestricted use, distribution, and reproduction in any medium, provided the original work is properly cited.

References

[1] Unnithan AKA, Mehta P. Hemorrhagic Stroke. Treasure Island (FL): StatPearls Publishing LLC; 2022

[2] Chen S, Zeng L, Hu Z. Progressing haemorrhagic stroke: Categories, causes, mechanisms and managements. Journal of Neurology. 2014;**261**(11):2061-2078

[3] An SJ, Kim TJ, Yoon BW. Epidemiology, risk factors, and clinical features of intracerebral Hemorrhage: An update. Journal of Stroke. 2017;**19**(1):3-10

[4] Karnath HO et al. The subcortical anatomy of human spatial neglect: Putamen, caudate nucleus and pulvinar. Brain. 2002;**125**(2):350-360. DOI: 10.1093/brain/awf032

[5] Talhatu HK et al. Clinical and demographic correlates of unilateral spatial neglect among community dwelling Nigerian stroke survivors. African Journal of Neurological Sciences. 2012;**31**(1)

[6] Plummer P, Morris ME, Dunai J. Assessment of unilateral neglect. Physical Therapy & Rehabilitation Journal. 2003;**83**:732-740

[7] Gammeri R et al. Unilateral spatial neglect after stroke: Current insights. Neuropsychiatric Disease and Treatment. Dovepress journal. 2020;**16**:131-152

[8] Sulay R, Sadhale A. Comparison of balance in sub-acute stroke patients with dominant lobe versus non-dominant lobe involvement of age group 25 to 60 years using balance evaluation system test (BESTest): A pilot study. International Journal of Health Sciences and Research. 2020;**10**(8):2249-9571. ISSN: 2249-957

[9] Di Monaco M, Schintu S, Dotta M, Barba S, Tappero R, Gindri P. Severity of unilateral spatial neglect is an independent predictor of functional outcome after acute inpatient rehabilitation in individuals with right hemispheric stroke. Archives of Physical Medicine and Rehabilitation. 2011;**92**:1250-1256

[10] Paolucci S, Antonucci G, Grasso MG, Pizzamiglio L. The role of unilateral spatial neglect in rehabilitation of right brain damaged ischemic stroke patients: A matched comparison. Archives of Physical Medicine and Rehabilitation. 2001;**82**:743-749

[11] Kimura Y et al. Impact of unilateral spatial neglect with or without cognitive impairments on independent gait recovery in stroke survivors. Journal of Rehabilitation Medicine. 2019;**51**(1): 26-31

[12] O'Sullivan SB, Schmitz TJ, Fulk GD. Physical Rehabilitation. Sixth ed. New Delhi: Jaypee Brothers Medical Publishers (P) Ltd; 2014. pp. 1235-1243

[13] Azouvi P et al. Rehabilitation of unilateral neglect: Evidence-based medicine. Annals of Physical and Rehabilitation Medicine. 2017;**60**:191-197

[14] Bowen A et al. Reasons for variability in the reported rate of occurrence of unilateral spatial neglect after stroke. Stroke. 1999;**30**:1196-1202

[15] Schroder ST et al. Clinical and functional differences between right and left stroke with and without contralateral spatial neglect. Journal of Rehabilitation Medicine. 2020;**52**:jrm0000X

[16] Saevarsson S, Kristjansson A, Hjaltason H. Unilateral neglect: A review

of causes, anatomical localization, theories and interventions. PubMed.gov National Library of Medicine. 2009;**95**(1):27-33

[17] Marques CLS et al. Validation of the Catherine Bergego scale in patients with unilateral spatial neglect after stroke. Dementia e Neuropsychologia. 2019;**13**(1):82-88

[18] Gammeri R et al. Unilateral spatial neglect after stroke: Current insights. Neuropsychiatric Disease and Treatment. Dovepress Journal. 2020;**16**:131-152

[19] Su C-Y et al. Neuropsychological impairment after hemorrhagic stroke in basal ganglia. Archives of Clinical Neuropsychology. 2007;**22**:465-474

[20] Bhatia KP, David Marsden C. The behavioural and motor consequences of focal lesions of the basal ganglia in man. Brain. 1994;**117**:859-876

[21] Hochstenbach et al. Congnitive deficits following stroke in basal ganglia. Scopus preview. Clinical Rehabilitation. 1998;**12**(6):514-520

[22] Mijovic-Prelec D, Bentley P, Caviness VS Jr. Selective rotation of egocentric spatial representation following right putaminal hemorrhage. Neuropsychologia. 2004;**42**:1827-1837

[23] Harris IM, Harris JA, Caine D. Mental-rotation deficits following damage to the right basal ganglia. Neuropsychology. 2002;**16**:524-537

[24] Coughlan AK. Effects of localised cerebral lesions and dysphasia on verbal memory. Journal of Neurology, Neurosurgery, and Psychiatry. 1979;**42**:914-923

Chapter 6

Neurofunctional Intervention Approaches

Joseph Nshimiyimana, Potien Uwihoreye, Jean Claude Muhigirwa and Theogene Niyonsega

Abstract

Neurofunctional approaches play the paramount functions in management of neurological disorders to improve the functional capability after impairments and activity limitations. These interventional approaches aligned with the neuroplasticity theories and all rely on repetition matters to build up engrams for the change of the brain function and activity performance. Affolter approach guides cognitive perceptual interaction through tactile-kinesthetic inputs. Neuromuscular facilitation relays the periphery information to the central nervous system by joint and muscle stimulus by using different techniques such stretching, irradiation, traction and approximation. Neurodevelopmental therapy manages the abnormal movement and postures through hands on facilitation of normal movement and inhibiting abnormal patterns movement. Roods approaches focus on the primitive reflexes through sensory stimuli to the targeted sensory receptors to initiate the appropriate motor pattern development. Brunnstrom approaches build on the synergies to provoke the engagement of the affected limbs. Task-oriented approaches are based on motor learning and involve repeat training with task-oriented activities. It is effective for improvement of the functional performance. It is a training method for encouraging functional movement with an interesting task. And also it improved the dexterity when applied using mixed interventions in hemiplegic.

Keywords: neurology, function, approaches, interventions, neurofunctions

1. Introduction

In 1980s, neurofunctional approaches (NFA) were presented as one of the few intercessions made fundamentally for clients with extreme shortfalls taking after traumatic brain injury (TBI) [1, 2]. Particularly, NFA is intended for clients who were restricted in their capacity to unravel novel issues or generalize abilities from one setting to another [3], and whose lack of insight constrained their capacity to engage within the rehabilitative process [3, 4]. This unit will summarize different approaches utilized as an interventional program for individuals enduring from distinctive neurological disorders.

2. Affolter approach

The Affolter approach is an innovative perceptual-cognitive approach developed in Switzerland by Felicie Affolter in 1981. Affolter holds the degrees in child psychology, education of normal, deaf, and language disordered children; audiology; and language pathology and speech sciences [5]. She studied with Jean Piaget and uses his interaction model of development as a foundation for her theory. Affolter and Walter Biscofberger have conducted research specifically involving development based on tactile-kinesthetic (T-K) interaction. Affolter theory and treatment approach is designed to give the student food for thought about the process of cognitive-perceptual development and the relationship that exists between T-K input and problem-solving skills in daily life [6]. This practical technique emphasizes evaluation and treatment in realistic situations using functional and age-appropriate activities. It has been successfully used in the treatment of coma recovery; cerebral vascular accident (CVA), TBI, and other neurological deficits including Alzheimer's disease and aging issues, pervasive developmental disorder and autism, and learning disabilities [5]. The Affolter concept challenges the clinician to take a hands-on functional approach in the treatment of T-K perceptual deficits in addition to using the standard evaluations and assessment for visual and auditory perceptual processing. Affolter has developed the treatment technique of nonverbal guiding to facilitate perceptual-cognitive interaction. Therapy is geared toward emphasizing appropriate input through a problem-solving process rather than focusing on the output and successful completion of a product. In using this treatment technique, specific guideline should be carefully followed and continually practiced.

2.1 Assumptions about the treatment framework

2.1.1 Treating patients in real situations

A fundamental assumption of treatment is that children with Pervasive Developmental Disorder (PDD) do have the ability to learn, and adults with acquired brain damage can relearn, but they require offer of assistance in doing so [7, 8]. To provide them with the assistance, we must help them organize in the way they search information in a better way, so that interaction improves, and the root can grow [9]. Organizing the seek for data requires identifying sources of data and isolating significant [10], from unessential sources when interacting and participate in activities with a therapist's hand to guide the patient makes a significant change [10, 11]. To achieve this goal, patients need intervention in actual daily life situations, not in artificial environments.

2.1.2 Targeting change in the underlying system

The work of this therapy does not intend the specific skills as a separate skill or isolated goals of treatment that are separated from the interaction of tasks solving problems in everyday life [12]. If the child cannot eat or participate in play properly, treatment does not pay attention on the same principles [13], that is, enabling nonverbal interactions to occur by enabling the patient to pick up adequate information for interacting with the environment around them [13, 14]. Visual or auditory inputs are not presumed to be of adequate information, rather a tactile perception [15]. The input that is viewed as essential and primary is tactile input [16]. In the absence of tactile information, to help patients, treatment must be designed to get this information [17]. However, to get these inputs are not from the outside environment for participating in everyday life [15, 17]. The kind and quantity of the data available for interaction are regarded as context dependent [18]; the situation demands changes from time to time and specifically with the required information for interaction [18]. Therefore, interacting in the activity is seen in the way of problem-solving event in all its aspects [19], including evaluating the processes, testing and creating in everyday life (for-example; eating spaghetti from the plate, getting toys from bathtub, putting on shoes, and getting a package through the door [20]. The problem to be solved or not will depend on the situation and available information in that situation [21].

3. Proprioceptive neuro-muscular facilitation

What we know nowadays as proprioceptive neuromuscular help (PNF) started as "proprioceptive assistance" a term created by Dr. Herman Kabat in the early 1940s. In 1954, Dorothy Voss included the word "neuromuscular" to deliver us the presently familiar proprioceptive neuromuscular facilitation, (PNF) [22]. Dr. Kabat's conceptual system for PNF came from his encounter as a neurophysiologist and doctor [23]. The work of Elizabeth Kenney, an Australian nurse who treated polio patients with particular stretching and strengthening exercises, was an early impact on Kabat [24]. Kenny's work was seen as a flight from the typical treatment at the time but needed the establishing of the sound neurophysiological method of reasoning Kabat coordinates Sister Kenney's manual method with Sherrington's disclosure of progressive acceptance, corresponding innervation, and restraint, and the marvel of irradiation [22]. They conclusively stated that PNF is a neurophysiological approach in which impulses from the periphery are facilitated to the central nervous system (CNS) through the stimulation of sensory receptors present in muscles and around the joints by stretch, resistance, traction, approximation, and audiovisual. Many therapists use PNF to help people regain their range of motion after injury or surgery [25]. However, it can also be used by athletes and dancers to improve their flexibility [26].

3.1 Principles of proprioceptive neuromuscular facilitation

The effectiveness of the PNF principles and procedures based on the integration of the appropriate use of joint and soft tissues mobilization [25]. The core PNF science can be universally utilized in any treatment approach [26], since the foundation is the evaluation and treatment of posture and movement [27]. The utilization of PNF for spinal dysfunction is enhanced by different working knowledge such as arthrokinematics, neurophysiology, and possible pathomechanics of the spine [27].

1. All Human beings have potentials that are not fully developed: Motor activity is restricted to the individual's physical capacity and characteristic and already learned neuromuscular reactions [28]. In any case, the typical individual incorporates a tremendous and undiscovered neuromuscular potential, which may be created through natural impacts and deliberate choices or tapped amid upsetting scenes [29, 30]. Through the use of client's strengths; the patient is motivated to achieve high level of function to minimize his or her weaknesses according to this philosophy [31].

2. Cephalocaudal and proximal distal is a normal motor development direction: Head, and neck develops first and then the trunk and lastly, in the extremities [32]. Proximal to distal points is a way of motor development [32]. Amid thera-

py, the neck and head are considered first during treatment since they affect the design of the motion in the body [26]. As well the next motor development is the trunk, which has central role of the body alignment [27]. Fine motor skills and extremities are developed following optimal function of the head and neck [26].

3. Reflex activity is dominant factor in early motor behavior [33]. Mature motor behavior is supported by postural reflex mechanisms; in therapy, weak muscles are supported through the facilitation of reflexes and by choosing developmental posture [33], functional activity initiation, or entailing trunk and head with extremity patterns [34].

4. Shifts between flexors and extensors dominance, are the cyclic trends evidenced during the growth of motor behavior [34]. Amid the useful action, movement flexion and extension changes [34]. This relationship is a complement that results to balance of postures and steadiness [34]. Facilitating reciprocal relationship of flexors and extensors reestablishes balance and stability during treatment [35].

5. Reversed actions make up activities that are regarded as goal-directed: rhythmic and reversing actions referred to as normal [36]. To establish balance among activities reversing movements are necessary and this brings balance and interaction between antagonists [36]. To enhance functioning, therapy must encourage movement in both directions [36].

6. Both balanced interaction of antagonists, normal posture, and movement depend on "Synergism" [34]; the balance of flexor dominance, movement reversal, and balance of reflex activity provide functional movement [34, 36]. During therapy sessions, in-equilibrium in these factors, to restore normal patterns of motion and posture responses are corrected [35]. Achieving these motor functions is through transitions between postures; such functions are doing reciprocal tasks, rolling, prone to supine or from sitting [37].

7. Total patterns of movement and posture are developed in a sequence to develop motor behavior [30]; specific sequence is followed during the development of motor behavior [30]. During development, complex functions are developed by early developmental milestones [30, 37]. The progress of motor behavior is in an orderly manner from mobility to stability to controlled mobility and into function [24], and developed an adverse repertoire of motor behavior [24]. Combined movements of the neck, trunk, and extremities also progress in a specified sequence [38].

4. Rood approach

Rood's approach is one of the neurophysiological and traditional approach based on hierarchical theories of CNS development [39]. This approach was developed by Margaret Rood in 1940 [40]. The essential concepts of this approach involves the motor patterns development through the sensory stimuli based on primitive reflexes and normal motor development patterns to progress motor performance skills [41, 42]. Rood's approach theories support the activation and de-activation of the receptors by sensory stimulation through facilitation and inhibition techniques [41]. Which of them concerned with the interaction of different factors such somatic, psychic and motor behaviors regulations [42]. The roods approach used by different health professionals in handling the motor control problems of patients, resulted from neurological insults [43]. The interventions process of the approach is based on development of the CNS, whereby the motor pattern development facilitated or inhibited for rehabilitation purposes [44–46]. Rood's philosophy focused on establishing typical motor development through building up required motor engrams [47].

4.1 Rood's approach techniques

The key principles of the Rood approach includes: normalizing tone, sequential developmental of autogenic motor patterns, repetition and purposeful-directed movement [48]. Though Rood's theories started in the 1940s, todays there are few corrections experienced some time recently she passed on, the modification handle has proceeded till presently based on current neuroscientific evidence [41]. Margret Rood during the discovery of this approach, Rood developed stages of motor control: Mobility, stability, controlled mobility, and skill [49]. She further worked on the sequence of motor development during the development of a child under each stage; reciprocal inhibition, [50] innervation/mobility, a reflex governed by spinal and supraspinal centers, subserves a protective function [50], phasic and reciprocal type of movement [50], contraction of agonist and antagonist, co-contraction, [50] c0-innervation/stability, simultaneous agonist and antagonist contraction with antagonist supreme [50], heavy work/controlled mobility [50], Stockmeyer "mobility superimposed on stability", and Creeping [50]. Skill, crawling, walking, reaching, activities requiring the coordinated use of hands [49, 50]. Rood's approach is one of several of the neurophysiological approaches created at that time and is centered upon four fundamental concepts to consider amid treatment: duality, the ontogenetic sequence, manipulation of the autonomic nervous system, and the level of sensitivity of the front horn cell [51, 52]. Following proprioceptive facilitatory techniques are used: heavy joint compression, stretch, intrinsic stretch, secondary ending stretch, stretch pressure, resistance, tapping, vestibular stimulation, inversion, therapeutic vibration and osteo-pressure [45, 53]. Finally, she developed following spasticity; inhibitory technique: gentle shaking or rocking, slow stroking, slow rolling, light joint compression, tendinous pressure, maintained stretch and rocking in developmental stages [53].

5. Brunnstrom approach

In 1951, Dr. Thomas Twitchell, a neurologist, published a seminal paper in which he described the longitudinal progression of motor recovery in 121 patients [54]. Twitchell observed that, early in recovery, these people tended to demonstrate stereotypical movement patterns. In addition, he observed that they tended to progress in their motor recovery through a consistent series of stages [54]. Twitchell did not hypothesize why some patients recovered further than others and did not present any recommendations for therapeutic interventions that might influence motor recovery [55]. Signe Brunnstrom, a physical therapist, combined Twitchell's findings with her own clinical observations to develop a treatment approach that was designed to facilitate the progression through the stages of recovery that Twitchell had reported. Brunnstrom's major contributions were:

- Her detailed description of reflexes and associated reactions exhibited by patients with post-stroke hemiplegia

- The concept of flexor and extensor synergy patterns in the paretic arm and leg
- A postulated sequence of treatment, designed to move patents through seven stages of recovery for the arm and hand

Many of Brunnstrom's contributions remain influential today. The associated reactions and reflexes she described are still recognized as characteristic features of motor behavior in stroke survivors with limited recovery [56]. A major difference is that Brunnstrom advised therapists to use techniques to elicit these pathological responses in an effort to stimulate movement. Today, however, rehabilitation professionals seek to prevent eliciting these responses [46]. The current understanding is that reflexive movements are not precursors to active, functional motor performance. Currently, rehabilitation professionals disagree on whether to consider the limb synergies as primary sequelae of the neurological damage (as Brunnstrom and Twitchell stipulated) that patients develop when they attempt to move in spite of underlying mechanical obstacles, such as immobility at the pelvis or scapular [57]. Those who view the flexor and extensor synergies of the upper limb as maladaptive strategies organize therapeutic interventions to prevent or remove specified "obstacles to movement" that may lead the person to develop inefficient motor strategies. Those who view the synergies as unavoidable motor deficits that precede full recovery of motor function are not concerned when patients move in these stereotypical patterns of movement [57]. There is no controversy, however, about the efficacy of following a therapeutic sequence in which the therapist guides the patient in moving through the six postulated stages of recovery. This paradigm for structuring motor therapy is not supported by current understanding of neuroplasticity and recovery of motor function after stroke.

5.1 Brunnstrom stages of recovery for the affected arm

According to [58], in their study on a neurophysiological and clinical study of Brunnstrom recovery stages in the upper limb following stroke, outlined the following stages of motor recovery:

Stage I Flaccidity: no voluntary movement, muscle tone, or reflexive responses
Stage II Synergies can be elicited reflexively; spasticity is developing
Stage III Beginning voluntary movement but only in synergy; spasticity may be significant
Stage IV Spasticity begins to decrease; ability to voluntarily perform movements that deviate slightly from synergy patterns
Stage V Increased control of isolated voluntary movements, independent of synergy patterns
Stage VI Isolated motor control; spasticity is minimal
Stage VII Normal speed and coordination of motor function

5.2 Principles of the Brunnstrom approach

The Brunnstrom approach is based on two key principles: Principle both normal movement which signifies how a healthy individual moves, [59] it requires muscles to work together, following damage to the CNS the muscles will not work as well together [59–61]. During recovery, muscles will start working together better and following damage to the CNS, movement recovery follows a specific sequence [59, 61]. The sequence is:

- There may be no "voluntary" movement after immediate onset of the injury.
- Spasticity appears, and basic movement reflexes occur.
- Patient begins to get voluntary control over their reflexes. This may leads to an increase in tone.
- Basic motor movement patterns are developed. This leads to a reduction in increase in tone (spasticity). Thus the complex motor movement patterns are learned and there's a remarkable decreasing in tone.
- Spasticity vanishes and individual movements mastered and coordination skills advanced approximately normal and then normal function restored.

6. Neurodevelopmental therapy/Bobath approach

Bobath approach which is also known as neurodevelopmental treatment (NDT) [62], is named after a physiotherapist Berta Bobath, and her husband Karl, a neuropsychiatrist proposed it for management of neurological injury impairments [62]. The Bobath approach is defined as client-centered hands on and a problem-solving approach [63]. It is used in management of individuals with abnormal movement and postures resulted from neurological injuries [63, 64]. This approach was first developed for effective management of patients with cerebral palsy manifested by neuro-motor dysfunctions [65–67]. The Bobath concept provided a reference that viewed children with Cerebral Palsy (CP) as having difficulty with postural control and movement against gravity [50]. The Bobath concept provided a reference that viewed children with CP as having difficulty with postural control and movement against gravity [50]. Bobath approach is used in all age group of persons with CNS lesion which resulted into functional dysfunction either movement of postural control. It is referred as both problem-solving approach to the assessment and treatment [68]. This approach underpinned the neurophysiological theories of motor control, motor learning and neural plasticity. This relied on new normal movement patterns and postures learned as a result mastered, and forms cortical representation of repetitive motor patterns. According to [69], the functional movement needs motor, sensory, cognitive, perceptual and biomechanical to be well efficiently produced in individuals with neurological injury. The task learning is influenced by the environmental condition, performance components needed to perform an activity and the evidence showed that neurofacilitation techniques of handling increases sensorimotor in initiation and performing the activity [70].

6.1 Clinical approach of Bobath concept

6.1.1 Motor control

Bobath approach concerns with personal factors such as sensory, perception, adaptive behavior and motor control skills of patient [71]. Bobath approach which is task-specific and goal-directed approach, [72] facilitates the optimal motor functions of the individual through the organization of proprioceptive and exteroceptive environments [72]. This client-centered approach focuses on neurological impairments resulted from either UMNL or LMNL to change motor performance [73], through selective activation of cutaneous and muscle receptors [63]. The muscle activation and sensory input to specific task facilitates complete accomplishment of the task in different contexts and environments, [74] taking into account the perceptual and cognitive demands [74]. It is recommended to be practiced in different real-life situation other than clinical milieu [23].

6.2 Basic principles of Bobath approach/neurodevelopmental treatment

According to [75], there are six principles of NDT management:

- Individualize functional outcomes: Interventions should consist of activities and strategies specific to the patient's needs, based on both the patient's unique limitations and his/her functional goals.

- Emphasis on motor control: Choose the therapeutic activities that encourage the client's active participation in order to promote both problem-solving and active use of muscles. This means getting past the redundant use of omni-cycle or a Nu-step. The activities should be meaningful to the patient as well as give them a chance to learn a novel movement [76].

- Increase active use of the affected or involved side: Find opportunities to involve the affected side in intervention activities, even if this means filing in the movement gaps with physical handling techniques.

- Provide practice: Allow the patient to practice and repeat activities in order to refine and recover movement.

- Teach 24-hour management: As mentioned previously, provide education in order to carry over learned tasks during therapy to other parts of the patient's day.

- Use and interdisciplinary approach: Involve all relevant rehabilitation disciplines (OT, PT and SLP) and ensure the carryover of NDT techniques.

A case scenario of application of Bobath approach in training sitting and standing. They are both main motor function to achieve independent locomotion, to use upper limb and hand [77]. In daily life of individuals these activities of sitting and standing acts as the major in performing other activities including normal movement, locomotion, reaching and grasping [78]. They are a number of different factors which influence the training of sit to stand including seat height, foot positon and upper limb. Seat height, the research evidence considered the length of levers in individuals but the modification and adaption is important respectively the capacity of the patient to optimize progressively the performance of the patients and also grading down or up is considered as the patient is improving the performance capacity [79–81]. Foot position has the impact in sitting to standing positons. During the initiation of the propulsion the heels should be either up or down, even it has limited number of researches and need more discussion [82]. The several studies support the position of the upper limb should be folded across the body. The position facilitated lower limb propulsion [83]. Interlimb neural coupling support the body alignment and proper activity activation as the major the concept of Bobath approach. In addition it releases the workloads of the lower limb [79]. According to [83] the restriction of upper limb in involvement of the body postural transition from sitting to standing remarkably changes the nature of the task. The study conducted [84] mentioned four core stages of sitting to stand namely flexion momentum, momentum transfer, extension, and stabilization. Flexion momentum begins with initiation of the movement and ends just before the buttocks lift from the chair (seat off). Momentum transfer begins at seat off and ends at maximal ankle dorsiflexion. Extension phase just after maximal ankle dorsiflexion until cessation of hip extension. Stabilization from when hip extension ceases until all movement has stopped.

As described in **Table 1** there are many factors which have to be taken into consideration when implementing this approach and evaluating its outcome and effectiveness. The mentioned aspect can have an influence in achieving the goal with the patient. Thus when choosing the task, the therapist need to think of multiple varieties in terms of task nature, person capacity and environmental contexts.

During interventions the nature of therapy based on task demands, impairments and environmental contexts as shown in **Table 2**.

Task/goal	individual	Environment
Sit to walk	Physical appearance	Clutters, unfriendly equipment, small space
Dressing	Ability of maintaining dynamic and static balance	
Transfer between seats	Perceptual and spatial awareness ability	For instance differences in height of seat, depth stability, arm supports, comparison with other materials such as a table or desk.
Stand to reach	Ability of flexibility	
STS while using upper	Age	
limb functionally	Pain	

Source: Schenkman et al. [84]·

Table 1.
Different aspects of the task, person and environment.

Task	Specific impairments	Environment
Task	Reduced ROM in the ankle for appropriate foot placement	Contextual practice
Practice		Adaptability of the environment to facilitate the task
Repetition	Reduced trunk alignment for weight transfer	
Variation		
Timing	Postural activity in low toned upper limb	
Speed and range		
Grade up and down		
The demands and performance of the task		
Challenging the use of cognition		
Dual tasking		
Contexts		

Source: Schenkman et al. [84].

Table 2.
Components of therapy setting to be considered.

7. Constrained induced movement therapy

Constrained Induced Movement Therapy (CIMT) showed the effective improvement in post-stroke patient improving the motor function of the affected arm [85]. This approach forced the affected arm to involve in task-oriented activities such as Activities of Daily Living (ADLs) [85]. Transcranial magnetic stimulation showed the increase in electrical stimulation on lesioned area from pre-to post Constrained Induced (CI) therapy to patient with stroke. There is expansion of the motor cortex representation of the affected arm. The cortical reorganization remarkably increased in mental imaging of the motor functional activities being repeated by the affected arm [86, 87]. In acute post-stroke patients there was a high significance improvement in all scores of Barthel index and functional independence measure (FIM) measures (eating, bathing, grooming and dressing) [88]. The intervention provided is the application of padded mitten on unaffected arm and training an affected arm with UE motor function and ADLs for at least 6 hours/day during 14 days [88]. This is the similar protocol that was first developed by Taub [86, 89] in investigation of the effects of CIMT on humans. However the protocol different from Taub referred to as modified CIMT (mCIMT). CIMT has high effects on affected upper limb of the stroke patients compared to other alternatives treatment or no treatment. This approach of CIMT work in more neurological conditions including spinal cord injury [90], where the study conducted on effects to Unilateral cortical Spinal Tract Injury in adults rat prove that there was growth and synapse formation of CST fibers from the intact side into the denervated spinal cord, synapse formation in the denervated cervical gray matter [90]. Growth and arborization of CST fibers was accompanied by marked behavioral improvements. But not limited to other conditions such as Multiple Sclerosis and cerebral palsy [90–94].

8. Task-oriented approach

Task-oriented approach found as an important approach in improving the functional outcomes in post-neurological injured persons. There was proved that balance, ADLs, and self-efficacy improved in hemiplegic patients [95, 96]. The provided interventions done in five times a week for four weeks, the session has 30 min, each task is performed three times for 10 min, with a 2-min break between each task [97]. The evaluation tools were modified Barthel index, Berg balance scale, and self-efficacy scale. The results of the Mann-Whitney U test also revealed significant differences in the BBS, MBI, and SES scores before and after training ($p < 0.01$). This approach showed also a remarkable impact in improving the balance and upper body skills in children with cerebral palsy as the study conducted [98–100] proved that all subjects had positive changes in gaining stability of standing and walking. The interventions program provided in two times/week, 40 min/session during 15 weeks. The outcome of the intervention program is associated with the intelligence of the subjects that should be positive or negative respectively the level of the capacity to follow instructions and cognitive learning ability. The above client-centered task-oriented approach program was used as it is based on motor learning and involves repeat training with task-oriented activities [98].

The client-centered task-oriented approach program in **Table 3** was used, [98] and it is based on motor learning and involves repeat training with task-oriented activities [98]. It is effective for improvement of the functional performance of a child with CP [98]. In addition, it is a training method for encouraging functional movement while providing children with an interesting task [98]. And also it improved

Active region		Program
Vestibular set	Hammock	Turning away side to side hammock activities
	Swing	Lying on sway board turning away side to side
		Quoits game activity
	Roll	Roll side to side on roll
Therapy ball		Lying on therapy ball and roll
		sit on ball and bounce
Sway board activities		Lying down to keep balance
Standing activities		Sway board activities of standing and sitting
		Weight bearing
		walking with a bar support
		Walk while holding balance beam supports
		Spinning activity
Mat based activities		Movement (pushing a ball) standing up
Proprioceptive input activities		Standing, walking
		Joint movement
		Muscular strength

Source: Kim and Lee [98].

Table 3.
Task-oriented activities in children with cerebral palsy.

the dexterity when applied using mixed interventions in hemiplegic Cerebral palsy patient both bilateral manipulation and unilateral task-oriented activities [101, 102]. This approach preliminary study concluded that it should also be feasible and safe to be applied in persons with multiple sclerosis with moderate mobility impairments [103, 104]. The rigorous systematic review concluded that there is a little significance in improving the upper limb function and hand dexterity in patients with spinal cord injury thus the primary research was recommended for further re-evaluation of the effectiveness of the approach [105].

9. Mirror therapy

Mirror therapy is a motor imagery process that modulates central mechanisms of motor recovery and neural plasticity. Mirror Therapy (MT) might have an effect on premotor and somatosensory cortex to activate the neurons in facilitating motor functions [106, 107]. MT is implemented by asking the patient to sit in front of the table with mirror and putting the arms both affected and unaffected on different sides of the mirror and during the performing the activities with unaffected arm the patient looks at the mirror to form motor image. With a case scenario which provided a session of 20 min/day, 5 days/week for 4 weeks showed significance in improving motor function of upper extremity [108].

The findings of the clinical stated the good outcome in reducing motor impairments, motor functions and ADLs as they were examined by FIM, Brunnstrom stages of recovery and Fugl-Meyer assessment (FMA) [109–111]. The study combined MT and electronic-mesh-glove found higher significance in normalizing muscle tone, improving hand skills, transfer as they were examined by MAS, box and block test (BBT), Action Research Arm Test (ARAT), and FIM [112]. Both involves in use of sensory stimulation such as kinesthetic inputs and visual illusion. As mentioned before MT activates premotor and somatosensory cortex and MG influence the activation of the sensory motor cortex [113–115]. Thus there is an increase in stimulation of somatosensory inputs which is likely to have remarkable effect of MT on movement control recovery.

10. Interaction of person, occupation, and environment in activity participation after neurological disorder

10.1 Introduction

As neurological disorders occur to persons from different professions, the Neurorehabilitation team encounters the challenge of helping clients in returning to a vast variety of occupations. These occupations include the different fields such as business, law, maintenance, office work, terrain work, medicine, housekeeping, accounting, police work, and as well as self-care occupations. Those challenges are grouped into three main aspects; which are person, occupation, and environmental. The quality of a person's experience, with regards to their level of satisfaction and functioning, is the outcome of the fit between the person-environment-occupation transactions [116].

10.2 Changes at person level after neurological disorder

After neurological disorder occurs to person level; there are changes in sensory and motor function, cognitive components, volition (interest and values), and financial; those changes interfere activity participation in many ways.

i. Sensory and motor function: It involves two types of symptoms: "negative" and "positive" sensory phenomena [117]. A phenomenon in which there are deficits in sensation such as hyperalgesia, is called negative symptoms [117]. However, a positive sensory phenomenon means the abnormal increase of functional sensation such paresthesia or neuropathic pain [117].

ii. Cognitive components: Cognitive impairment and memory loss are common after a stroke. Stroke affects the cognitive domain, which includes attention, memory, language, and orientation [117]. The most affected domains are attention and executive functions; at the time of stroke diagnosis, memory problems are often prominent, the presence of well-functioning cognitive skills is the cornerstone of occupational engagement.

iii. Volition: It includes the thoughts and feelings about personal capacity and effectiveness and how a person perceives the importance of what they do as well as what bring them enjoyment and satisfaction [118]. Neurological disorders disrupt participation in some interests that require the use of body structure, body function, and social engagement at home and outside of the home. A sudden inability to act on one's volition is likely to lead to a decreased quality of life [119]. Not being able to participate in challenging and enjoyable work tasks or leisure activities will erode one's feelings of self-efficacy and sense of personal capacity.

10.3 Environment: impact of occupational, social, and physical environment

Neurological disorders do not only affect person internally but also environment, therefore creating a need to modify environment to support their interests and roles. The MOHO classifies environment into three components: Physical, social, and occupational environment [120]. The physical environment includes both natural and built space where people do their day-to-day activities, changes due to neurological disorders. People who work at home or from home are required to find a supportive space at home or outdoor for participating in day-to-day activities. Occupational environment: According to Black [121], Occupational environment may be defined as the workplace surroundings that encompass the physical and social environment. The social environment can be seen as social relationships, immediate physical surroundings and cultural settings in which people function and interact. The patient with neurological disorders experiences a number of environment barriers, limiting their participation and re-integration after being discharged from hospital. Social environment: The social attitudes define the big part in participation of different areas of engagement such as education, employment, health care and public realm [122]. Negative attitudes towards the persons with disability hinder them from exploring their potentialities like other persons without disability. However, the positive social attitudes enhance the participation in more than one area [122]. Among of them includes home and community based engagement and inclusion, which in turn strengthen self-esteem through sense of belonging [122].

10.4 Applying person-environment-occupation model interventions post neurological disorders

Figure 1 shows the extent of congruence in the person-environment-occupation (PEO) relationships is represented by the degree of overlap between the three spheres; the closer the spheres overlap, the greater the degree of harmony or fit [123]. According to PEO, the environment influences both person and occupation but, more importantly it can be easily modified more than person [116]. Thus the fitting between person, occupation and environment depends on the adaptability between those three components respectively the achieving goal of person [116]. Activity, task and occupation are all interrelated as they are the intervention tools used to gain occupational performance.

11. Neuro-functional disorders assessment

11.1 Introduction

Functional neurological disorders (FND) are among the most common causes of neurological disability [124]. There is no single factor to consider the cause of FND, but rather a combination of factors interacting together [125]. The etiology of FND is still specifically not known [126]. FND is caused by a complex combination of biological, psychological and social factors on the brain [127]. Referring to Diagnostic and Statistical Manual of Mental Disorders, Fifth Edition (DSM-5) [128], the term

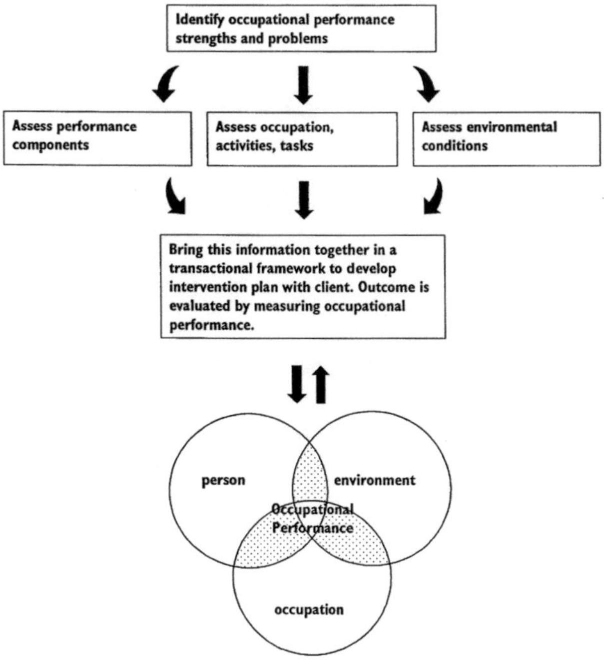

Figure 1.
Person-Environment-Occupation(PEO) relationship.

functional was adopted as the primary definition in the functional neurological symptom disorder [128]. This provides causative neutrality and may also increase patient understanding and acceptance [128]. The first decision in management of FND is the proper diagnosis followed by the explanation of the condition to the patients and care givers. After establishment of the disabling condition, rehabilitation team intervenes for long-term management [129]. Prior to individual follow up, every rehab personnel conduct a thorough assessment to highlight challenges to function and plan accordingly. The intervention plan should also include patient or caregiver involvement. Comorbidities, such as pain or fatigue and psychiatric comorbidities (anxiety, depression, dissociation etc.) should be carefully evaluated, as they need an individualized treatment plan [129].

11.2 Features of functional neurologic disorders

Motor FND, Suggestive clinical features include sudden onset, disappearance with distraction, increase with attention, and excessive fatigue or demonstration of effort [128]. With motor deficit, the presenting feature of the patients includes but not limited to dysfunctions of body structures in engagement of voluntary and purposeful task [130]. This includes inability to walk and to move the arm [125]. Sensation: sensory impairments in persons with neurological disorders include sensory loss, pain and abnormal sensation such as light touch and vibration [126]. The proprioceptive sensation mighty be also affected whereby the person losses the ability to sense the body part position [130]. Proprioception is tested by asking the patient to close eyes, and position the joint in space and let the patient identify the joint position [131]. A patient with functional proprioception will be able to correctly identify the exact placement of body part. Axial FND, Functional axial disturbances include disorders of gait and posture such as excessive gait slowness, astasia-abasia and knee buckling [128]. Speech FND, the patients with speech difficulties experiences challenges in verbal response to the incoming request (Broca's aphasia) and understanding instruction (expressive aphasia) [132].

11.3 Areas of assessment for neuro-functional deficits patients

This is where now practice makes good performance, neurological exam sounds intimidating in the first occasions but the more ones enroll into examination, the more proficient becomes [129]. This is a hands-on patient stage and should not be escaped whenever neurological disorder is suspected.

The neurological exam can be organized into seven categories:

1. mental status,
2. cranial nerves,
3. motor system,
4. reflexes
5. sensory system
6. coordination
7. station and gait.
8. simulated functional activities

The practitioner approach neurological exam systematically and make sure that there is no area left unevaluated so as to mark the proper prognosis [129]. The preference of assessment approach should be followed to compare the affected part vs normal, distal vs proximal and let vs right mores especially the sensory impairments [129]. Mental Status: The mental status defines the reliability of the rest of neuro-exam. The patient keeps the appropriate eye contact and does not need things repeated, it signifies that he/she can converse. Thus you proceed with medical history and recent event in consistent manner [129]. The mental screening examinations include seven areas, which are attention, orientation, speech fluency, comprehension, verbal response, high cognitive involvement and memory [132]. But the therapist needs to test the status of mood to screening out the presence of psychiatric conditions [132]. This acts screening examination before deciding to proceed with high mental functions. Cranial Nerves: The cranial nerves consist of nerves that exit through foramina in the skull, not necessarily nerves that originate in the brain [131]. Neurologic impaired patients impose difficulties to the prognosis and recovery of the victim [133]. Therefore, cranial nerve screening should be set mandatory [133]. Thus a thorough evaluation should be included in evaluation process. Motor Exam: When assessing motor function among FND patients, it is of the utmost valuable to first distinguish the whether the case is of the upper motor neuron lesion or lower motor neuron lesion [131]. Depending on the strength of the patient, motor evaluation may incorporate mobility [131]. During motor examination the practitioner is recommended to conduct motor exam to measure fall risk prior to evaluation to minimize the falling incidence [131]. Furthermore, during motor assessments the practitioners observes different aspects of person such as muscle build ups, muscle tone, endurance and movement [134]. As well both equilibrium and non-equilibrium tests should be considered whilst evaluating coordination deficits. In addition, the practitioner has to keep a limb in Position in such a way that there is risk of recruiting other muscles with similar function are kept minimal [135]. Reflexes: Tendon Reflex test is the most objective part of the neurological exam and is the least dependent on cooperation [131]. When test reflexes, the muscle for which tendon to be tested should be put to tension [131] and stress then quickly tap or use the standardized reflex or knee hammer to the tendon to be tested and observe the reaction [131]. The intensity and extent of briskness response has to be analyzed [131]. This should be repeated to the other side and compare against the normal range. Sensation: Both superficial and deep sensation should be tested in all four limbs. Superficial sensation (pain and temperature) this is channeled by unmyelinated and small myelinated nerve fibers through the ascending tract of spinothalamic [136]. Pain sensation can be tested with a safety pin or the broken end of a cotton swab [136]; temperature sensation can be tested with a hot or cold fluid filled test tubes [136], however cool metal object like a tuning fork maybe used as an alternative [136]. Deep sensation which combines pressure, proprioception, and vibration is mediated by large fibers through the dorsal and lateral aspects of the ascending tract [124]. Coordination and Gait Assessment: Incoordination should be noted when patient sits and stands upright, or getting onto the examination table [126]. Gait assessment should not be separated far from coordination among functional neurologic disorder patients [129]. Position of body in space, posture and extremity placement [137] and, speed, steadiness, arm swinging, heel strikes, stance, and heel to toe walking have to be considered in evaluation of gait [137]. While neurologists and other physicians play an important role early on, the treatment of FND, it is typically the purview of allied health professionals, including physical therapist, occupational therapist, speech and language pathologist, art, and recreational therapists to conduct assessment prior to intervention [130].

12. Conclusions

The neurofunctional interventional approaches imply the significant impact in changing the activity participation of persons with neurological disorder and injury in terms of treating impairments and improving the ability of activity performance after injury. These approaches have been approved by many clinical based evidences and they are mostly contextualized according to the nature of setting, nature of patient and therapist's own experience. Furthermore, among of all those traditional sensorimotor approaches have no remarkable significant difference in effectiveness and efficiency. Thus the therapist chooses the approach according to his/her experience in certain approach, clients conditions and practicing milieu. Besides to that all approaches favor the theories of neuroplasticity and building up required engrams needs repetitions. Apart from that the status of person, task and nature of real working environment have important influence in achieving the goal with the clients with neurological disorder or injury as long as brain insults result in many different areas of impairments such as motor, sensory, cognition and psychosocial issues.

Acknowledgements

NJ: Involved in reviewing articles and wrote about the literature of neurofunctional interventional approaches, involved in organizing and preparing the book chapter and followed up the progress of book chapter. UP: Involved in reviewing the articles and wrote about the literature of neurofunctional interventional approaches. NT: Involved in reviewing the articles and wrote about the literature of interaction of person, occupation, and environment in activity participation after neurological disorder. MJ: Involved in reviewing the articles and wrote about the literature of neurofunctional disorders assessment.

Conflict of interest

None declared.

Author details

Joseph Nshimiyimana[1*], Potien Uwihoreye[2], Jean Claude Muhigirwa[3] and Theogene Niyonsega[4]

1 Department of Occupational Therapy, Gahini Rehabilitation Center, Kayonza, Rwanda

2 Department of Occupational Therapy, King Faisal Hospital, Kigali, Rwanda

3 Department of Occupational Therapy, Autism Individual Care Center, Kigali, Rwaanda

4 Department of Occupational Therapy, Ndera Neuropsychiatric Hospital/Icyizere Branch, Kigali, Rwanda

*Address all correspondence to: josephnshimiyimana50@gmail.com

IntechOpen

© 2022 The Author(s). Licensee IntechOpen. This chapter is distributed under the terms of the Creative Commons Attribution License (http://creativecommons.org/licenses/by/3.0), which permits unrestricted use, distribution, and reproduction in any medium, provided the original work is properly cited.

References

[1] Koelsch S, Jacobs AM, Menninghaus W, Liebal K, Klann-Delius G, von Scheve C, et al. The quartet theory of human emotions: An integrative and neurofunctional model. Physics of Life Reviews. 2015;**13**:1-27

[2] Cerasa A, Gioia MC, Salsone M, Donzuso G, Chiriaco C, Realmuto S, et al. Neurofunctional correlates of attention rehabilitation in Parkinson's disease: An explorative study. Neurological Sciences. 2014;**35**(8):1173-1180

[3] Clark-wilson J, Giles GM, Baxter DM. Revisiting the neurofunctional approach: Conceptualizing the core components for the rehabilitation of everyday living skills. Brain Injury. 2014;**9052**:1646-1656

[4] Kose N, Muezzinoglu O, Bilgin S, Karahan S, Isikay I, Bilginer B. Early rehabilitation improves neurofunctional outcome after surgery in children with spinal tumors. Neural Regeneration Research. 2014;**9**(2):129-134

[5] DiFonzo N, Bordia P. Reproduced with permission of the copyright owner. Further reproduction prohibited without. Journal of Allergy and Clinical Immunology. 1998;**130**(2):556. DOI: 10.1016/j.jaci.2012.05.050

[6] Stockman IJ. Movement and Action in Learning and Development: Clinical Implications for Pervasive Developmental Disorders. American Psychological Association. 2004. Available from: https://psycnet.apa.org/record/2004-12472-000

[7] van de Rakt J, McCarthy-Grunwald S. Rehabilitation of the upper limb after an stroke. Part 2. Italian Journal of Sports rehabilitation and Posturology. 2021;**10**(22):2243-2277

[8] Nielsen AI, Power E, Jensen LR. Communication with patients in post-traumatic confusional state: Perception of rehabilitation staff. Brain injury. Mar 2020;**34**(4):447-455

[9] Andelic N, Bautz-Holter E, Ronning P, Olafsen K, Sigurdardottir S, Schanke AK, et al. Does an early onset and continuous chain of rehabilitation improve the long-term functional outcome of patients with severe traumatic brain injury? Journal of Neurotrauma. 2012;**29**(1):66-74

[10] McCabe P, Lippert C, Weiser M, Hilditch M, Hartridge C, Villamere J. Community reintegration following acquired brain injury. Brain Injury. 2007;**21**(2):231-257

[11] Goodman J, Hurst J, Locke C, editors. Occupational therapy for people with learning disabilities: a practical guide. Elsevier Health Sciences; Nov 2008

[12] Uys ME, Su BOT, Us MOT, Buchanan H, Uct OT. Return to work for people with hand injuries in South Africa: Occupational therapy strategies. South African Journal. 2020;**50**(2):52-61

[13] Resources H, White S, White S. Assessment and Treatment of Childhood Apraxia of Speech: The Perspective of Current Speech-Language Pathologists Speech-Language Pathologists. University of Arkansas, Fersity of Arkansa; May 2022;(3):8-17

[14] Vachel W, Friedrich W. Reproductions supplied by EDRS are the best that can be made from the original document. IDCA, Washington, DC. Bureau of Africa. Jun 2002;(4):034-191

[15] Pauff SM, Miller SC. Motor and tactile-perceptual skill differences between individuals with high-functioning autism and typically

developing individuals ages 50-21. Bone. 2012;**78**(2):711-716

[16] Marczak M, Ginszt M, Gawda P, Berger M, Majcher P. Neurocognitive functioning of sport climbers. Journal of Human Kinetics. 2018;**65**(1):13-19

[17] Naess HL, Vikane E, Wehling EI, Skouen JS, Bell RF, Johnsen LG. Effect of early interdisciplinary rehabilitation for trauma patients: A systematic review. Archives of Rehabilitation Research and Clinical Translation [Internet]. 2020;**2**(4):100070. DOI: 10.1016/j.arrct.2020.100070

[18] Barroso M. Workplace relationships in Europe: An analysis by occupation and employment status. Intangible Capital. 2022;**18**(1):39

[19] Maier M, Ballester BR, Verschure PFMJ. Principles of neurorehabilitation after stroke based on motor learning and brain plasticity mechanisms. 2019;**13**(December):1-18

[20] Redcay E, Schilbach L. Using second-person neuroscience to elucidate the mechanisms of social interaction. Nature Reviews Neuroscience. 2020;**20**(8):495-505. DOI: 10.1038/s41583-019-0179-4

[21] Kim MK, Cho JH, Jeong JH. Classification of Tactile Perception and Attention on Natural Textures from EEG Signals. In: 9th IEEE Int Winter Conf Brain-Computer Interface, BCI 2021. 2021

[22] Smedes F, Heidmann M, Schäfer C, Fischer N, Stępień A. The proprioceptive neuromuscular facilitation-concept; the state of the evidence, a narrative review. The Physical Therapy Review. 2016;**21**(1):17-31

[23] Mikołajewska E. Bobath and traditional approaches in post-stroke gait rehabilitation in adults. Biomedical Human Kinetics. 2017;**9**(1):27-33

[24] Godges JJ, Mattson-bell M, Thorpe D. Neuromuscular facilitation on glenohumeral external rotation and overhead reach. The Journal of Orthopaedic and Sports Physical Therapy. 2003;**33**(12):713-718

[25] Hindle K, Whitcomb T, Briggs W, Hong J. Proprioceptive neuromuscular facilitation (PNF): Its mechanisms and effects on range of motion and muscular function. Journal of Human Kinetics. 2012;**31**(1):105-113

[26] Sajedi H. Effect of PNF, ballistic and static stretching on the range of motion after sports injury surgery in football athletes. African Educational Research Journal. 2020;**8**(1):105-109

[27] Saliba VL, Johnson GS, Wardlaw CH. Proprioceptive neuromuscular facilitation. Williams & Wilkins editors. Rational Manual Therapies. Institute of physical art: physical art. 1993;243

[28] Shimura K, Kasai T. Effects of proprioceptive neuromuscular facilitation on the initiation of voluntary movement and motor evoked potentials in upper limb muscles. 2002;**21**:101-113

[29] Areeudomwong P, Buttagat V. Brazilian Journal of Proprioceptive neuromuscular facilitation training improves pain-related and balance outcomes in working-age patients with chronic low back pain: A randomized controlled trial ☆. Brazilian Journal of Physical Therapy [Internet]. 2019;**23**(5):428-436. DOI: 10.1016/j.bjpt.2018.10.005

[30] Arcanjo FL, Martins JVP, Moté P, Leporace G, Oliveira DA de, Sousa CS de, et al. Proprioceptive neuromuscular facilitation training reduces pain and disability in individuals with chronic low back pain: A systematic review and meta-analysis. Complementary Therapies in Clinical Practice. 2022;46(November 2021)

[31] Bae SS, RPT, MA, MPH. A study of proprioceptive neuromuscular facilitation principles. Journal of The Korean Society of Physical Medicine. 1993;**5**:109-114

[32] Choi YK, Nam CW, Lee JH, Park YH. The effects of taping prior to PNF treatment on lower extremity proprioception of hemiplegic patients. Journal of Physical Therapy Science. 2013;**25**(9):1119-1122

[33] Campbell M, Mckenzie JE, Sowden A, Katikireddi SV, Brennan SE, Ellis S, et al. Synthesis without meta-analysis (SWiM) in systematic reviews: Reporting guideline. 2020;1-6

[34] Caldwell CC, Petzinger GM, Jakowec MW, Cadenas E. Treadmill exercise rescues mitochondrial function and motor behavior in the CAG140 knock-in mouse model of Huntington's disease. Chemico-Biological Interactions. 2020;**315**

[35] Fathi S, Taghizadeh G, Azad A, Behzadipour S, Shams Hafshejani D, Zare A, et al. Effects of Upper Extremity Coordination Exercises Based on Fatigue Prediction on Upper Extremity Sensory-motor Functions in Chronic Stroke Survivors. Iranian Rehabilitation Journal. 10 Mar 2022;**20**(4):17-28

[36] Johnson GS, Johnson V, Miller RA, Rudzinski L, Welsome KM. The Functional Mobilization Approach. In: Wise CH, editors. Orthopaedic Manual Physical Therapy: From Art to Evidence. McGraw Hill; 2015. Available from: https://fadavispt.mhmedical.com/content.aspx?bookid=2154&sectionid=164768190 [Accessed August 20,2022]

[37] Rotenberg-Shpigelman S, Erez ABH, Nahaloni I, Maeir A. Neurofunctional treatment targeting participation among chronic stroke survivors: A pilot randomised controlled study. Neuropsychological Rehabilitation. 2012;**22**(4):532-549

[38] Beckers D, Buck M. PNF Basic Principles and Procedures for Facilitation. InPNF in Practice. Berlin, Heidelberg: Springer; 2021. pp. 17-35. DOI: 10.1007/978-3-662-61818-9_2

[39] Bordoloi K, Deka RS. Scientific reconciliation of the concepts and principles of rood approach. International Journal of Health Sciences and Research. 2018;**8**(9):225-234

[40] Bordoloi K, Res RD-IJHS. Scientific reconciliation of the concepts and principles of rood approach. ResearchgateNet [Internet]. 2018, 2018;**8**(9):225. Available from: https://www.researchgate.net/profile/Kuki-Bordoloi/publication/327751077_Scientific_Reconciliation_of_the_Concepts_and_Principles_of_Rood_Approach/links/5ba25389299bf13e603cb620/Scientific-Reconciliation-of-the-Concepts-and-Principles-of-Rood-Approach.pdf

[41] Sangam S, Naveed A, Athar M, Prathyusha P, Moulika S, Lakshmi S. International Journal of Health Sciences and Research. 2015;**5**(1):156-164

[42] Bordoloi K, Deka RS. Effectiveness of home exercise program with modified rood's approach on muscle strength in post cerebral haemorrhagic individuals of assam: A randomized trial. pesquisa.bvsalud. International Journal of Physiotherapy. 2019;**6**(5):231-239. Available from: https://pesquisa.bvsalud.org/portal/resource/pt/sea-205758

[43] Ankar P, Samal S, Vikrant, Kovela RK, Dagal R, Thimoty R. Effect of physiotherapy on hand rehabilitation in acute ischemic stroke survivor: A case report. Journal of Pharmaceutical Research International. 2022;**34**:28-32

[44] Stockmeyer SA. An interpretation of the approach of Rood to the treatment of neuromuscular dysfunction. American journal of physical medicine & rehabilitation. 1 Feb 1967;**46**(6):900-956

[45] Patel BR, Kadam N, Pawar P. Effect of Rood's approach in diabetic polyneuropathy. Biomedical Research. 2019;**30**(3):469-474

[46] Cano-De-la-cuerda R. Influential women in the field of neurological rehabilitation: A literature review. International Journal of Environmental Research and Public Health. 2022;**19**(3):1112

[47] Yadav V, Gera C, Yadav R. Evolution in hemiplegic management: A review. International Journal of Medical Science and Public Health. 2018;**8**(5):360-369

[48] Radomski MV, Trombly Latham AA. Occupational Therapy for Physical Dysfunction. 7th ed. Tokyo: Wolters Kluwer; 2014. p. 617

[49] Khan FR, Chevidikunnan MF, BinMulayh EA, Gaowgzeh RA. Physical therapists' perspectives on improving walking capacity in patients with stroke: A cross-sectional study from Saudi Arabia. Journal of Musculoskeletal & Neuronal Interactions. 2020;**20**(2):223-233

[50] Rutherford M, Maciver D, Johnston L, Prior S, Forsyth K. Development of a Pathway for Multidisciplinary Neurodevelopmental Assessment and Diagnosis in Children and Young People. Children. 11 Nov 2021;**8**(6):1033. DOI: 10.3390/children8111033

[51] Lazarus CL. The role of therapeutic exercises in the treatment of dysphagia 3 the role of therapeutic exercises in the treatment of dysphagia lingual strengthening and swallowing. American journal of Speech-language pathology. 2005;**7**(3):1-35

[52] Chen X, Liu F, Yan Z, Cheng S, Liu X, Li H, et al. Therapeutic effects of sensory input training on motor function rehabilitation after stroke. 2018;**97**(48):e13387

[53] Marathe DN, Kunde C, Ganvir SS. A comparative study between the immediate effects of tendinous pressure technique versus myofascial release in the reduction of spasticity: A cross over study. VIMS Journal of Physical Therapy. 2020;**2**(1):21-27

[54] Bhattacharjee K, Shou MK. Additive effects of brunnstrom approach in combination with mechanical vibration and mirror neuron training on upper limb function in patients with subacute stroke - a single blinded randomized controlled trial. IJRAMT. 2022;**3**(2):16-21

[55] Lentinga AT. Diversity in neurological physiotherapy: A content analysis of the brunnstrom/bobath. International Journal of Innovative Science and Research Technology. May 2019;(5):23-36

[56] Su TJ, Lo KL, Tsai JSH, Yeh WA, Kuo CF. A Brunnstrom stage evaluation system with fuzzy-accelerometer. Applied Sciences. 2019;**9**(18)

[57] Pandian S, Arya KN, Kumar V, Joshi AK. Synergy-Based Motor Therapy Inducing Favorable Changes in Motor Function Components among Poststroke Subjects: A Single-Group Study. Journal of Neurosciences in Rural Practice. 8 Mar 2022;**13**(7):261-269. DOI: 10.1055/s-0042-1743458

[58] Naghdi S, Ansari NN, Mansouri K, Hasson S. A neurophysiological and clinical study of Brunnstrom recovery

stages in the upper limb following stroke. Brain Injury. 2010;**24**(11):1372-1378

[59] Chen J-C. Progress in sensorimotor rehabilitative physical therapy programs for stroke patients. World Journal of Clinical Cases. 2014;**2**(8):316

[60] Mehrbod N, Vahed N, Ahmadi M, Yekkehpoor M. Comparison of the effects of physiotherapy alone and video game-based therapy plus physiotherapy on depression and muscle strength in post-stroke patients. Journal of MAR Neurology and Psychology. 2022;**4**(2):1-12

[61] Nagano K, Hori H, Muramatsu K. A comparison of at-home walking and 10-meter walking test parameters of individuals with post-stroke hemiparesis. Journal of Physical Therapy Science. 2015;**27**(2):357-359

[62] Gray C, Ford C. Bobath therapy for patients with neurological conditions: A review of clinical effectiveness, cost-effectiveness, and guidelines. Wiley interScience Discover Something great. 2018;**11**:1-26

[63] Kalaichandran K, Swarnakumari DP. Neuro developmental treatment (ndt) for cerebral palsy: A clinical study. International Journal of Innovative Science and Research Technology. 2019;**4**(5):33-34

[64] Reynolds S, Lane SJ, Richards L. Using animal models of enriched environments to inform research on sensory integration intervention for the rehabilitation of neurodevelopmental disorders. Clinical Medicine Insights: Paediatrics. 2010;**13**:1-11

[65] Palisano RJ, Di Rezze B, Stewart D, Rosenbaum PL, Hlyva O, Freeman M, et al. Life course health development of individuals with neurodevelopmental conditions. Developmental Medicine and Child Neurology. 2017;**59**(5):470-476

[66] Uyangk M, Bumin G, Kayghan H. Comparison of different therapy approaches in children with Down syndrome. Official journal of the Japan Pediatric Society. Feb 2003;**45**(1):68-73

[67] Desorbay T. A neuro-developmental approach to specific learning difficulties. International Journal of Nutrition, Pharmacology, Neurological Diseases. 2013;**3**(1):1

[68] Iles R, Davidson M. Physiotherapy diagnosis in clinical practice: A survey of orthopaedic certified specialists in the USA. Physiotherapy Research International. 2008;**11**(2):93-103

[69] Mayston MJ, Harrison LM, Stephens JA. A neurophysiological study of mirror movements in adults and children. Ann Neurol. 1999;**45**(5):583-594

[70] Miyai I, Yagura H, Oda I, Konishi I, Eda H, Suzuki T, et al. Premotor cortex is involved in restoration of gait in stroke. Annals of Neurology. 2002;**52**(2):188-194

[71] Chowdhury S, Chakraborty PP. Universal health coverage - there is more to it than meets the eye. Journal of Family Medicine and Primary Care. 2017;6(2):169-170

[72] Zanon MA, Pacheco RL, Latorraca CDOC, Martimbianco ALC, Pachito DV, Riera R. Neurodevelopmental treatment (bobath) for children with cerebral palsy: A systematic review. Journal of Child Neurology. 2019;**34**(11):679-686

[73] Veličkovíć TD. Basic principles of the neurodevelopmental treatment (NDT) - bobath. Paediatria Croatica, Supplement. 2002;**46**(1):163-168

[74] Kosel M. International Journal of Developmental Neuroscience. Neurodevelopmental disorders: From pathophysiology to novel therapeutic approaches. Apr 2022;**82**(3):277-285

[75] Bierman JC, Franjoine MR, Hazzard CM, Howle JM, Stamer M. Neuro-Develpmental Treatment: A Guide to NDT Practice. New York: Thieme Publishers; 2016

[76] Rao AK. Approaches to motor control dysfunction: An evidence-based review. Stroke Rehabilitation. Journal of stroke rehabilitation. 2015;**10**:348-359

[77] Lomaglio MJ, Eng JJ. Muscle strength and weight-bearing symmetry relate to sit-to-stand performance in individuals with stroke. Gait & Posture. 2005;**22**(2):126-131

[78] Dean CM, Channon EF, Hall JM. Sitting training early after stroke improves sitting ability and quality and carries over to standing up but not to walking: A randomised controlled trial. Australian Journal of Physiotherapy. 2007;**53**(2):97-102. DOI: 10.1016/S0004-9514(07)70042-9

[79] Benvenuti ÃF, Bimbi C, Stanhope SJ, Mazza C. Movement strategy in sit-to-stand performance. Journal of the American Geriatric Society. Oct 2004;**52**(10):1750-1754

[80] Yamada T, geriatrics SD-A of gerontology and, 2009 undefined. Relationships between ground reaction force parameters during a sit-to-stand movement and physical activity and falling risk of the elderly and a comparison of the. Archives of Gerontology and Geriatrics. Elsevier [Internet]. 2009;**48**(1). Available from: https://www.sciencedirect.com/science/article/pii/S0167494307002208

[81] Roy G, Nadeau S, Gravel D, Malouin F, McFadyen BJ, Piotte F. The effect of foot position and chair height on the asymmetry of vertical forces during sit-to-stand and stand-to-sit tasks in individuals with hemiparesis. Clinical Biomechanics. Elsevier [Internet]. 2006;**21**(6). Available from: https://www.sciencedirect.com/science/article/pii/S0268003306000283

[82] Raine S, Meadows L, Lynch-Ellerington M, editors. Bobath Concept: Theory and Clinical Practice in Neurological Rehabilitation. John Wiley & Sons; 9 May 2013. pp. 2077

[83] Carr JH, Gentile AM. The effect of arm movement on the biomechanics of standing up. Human Movement Science. 1994;**13**(2):175-193

[84] Schenkman M, Berger RA, Riley PO, Mann RW, Hodge WA. Whole-body movements during rising to standing from sitting. Physical Therapy. 1990;**70**(10):638-651

[85] Wolf L. Dose and timing in neurorehabilitation: Prescribing motor therapy after stroke. HHS Public Access. 2016;**14**(2):224-234

[86] Mark VW, Taub E, Morris DM. Neuroplasticity and constraint-induced movement therapy. Europa Medicophysica. 2006;**42**(3):269-284

[87] Schaechter JD, Kraft E, Hilliard TS, Dijkhuizen RM, Benner T, Finklestein SP, et al. Motor recovery and cortical reorganization after constraint-induced movement therapy in stroke patients: A preliminary study. The American Society of Neurorehabilitation. 2002;**16**(4):1-13

[88] Dromerick AW, Edwards DF, Hahn M, Otr MS. Therapy during acute rehabilitation reduce arm impairment after ischemic stroke? American Heart Association, Inc. 2000;**18**(3):2984-2988

[89] Hakkennes S, Keating JL. Constraint-induced movement therapy following stroke: A systematic review of randomised controlled trials. Australian

Journal of Physiotherapy [Internet]. 2005;**51**(4):221-231. DOI: 10.1016/S0004-9514(05)70003-9

[90] Y-J Kim, J-K Kim, S-Y Park. Effects of modified constraint-induced movement therapy and functional bimanual training on upper extremity function and daily activities in a patient with incomplete spinal cord injury: A case study. Journal of Physical Therapy Science. 2015;**27**(12):3945-3946

[91] Mark VW, Taub E, Bashir K, Uswatte G, Delgado A, Bowman MH, et al. Constraint-induced movement therapy can improve hemiparetic progressive multiple sclerosis. Preliminary Findings. 2008;**14**(7):992-994

[92] Gordon AM, et al. Bimanual training and constraint-induced movement therapy in children with hemiplegic cerebral palsy: A randomized trial. Neurorehabilitation and neural repair. 2011;**25**(8):692-702

[93] Mark VW, et al. Phase II randomized controlled trial of constraint-induced movement therapy in multiple sclerosis. Part 1: Effects On Real-World Function. Neurorehabilitation and neural repair. 2018;**32**(3):223-232

[94] Mark VW. Constraint-induced movement therapy for the lower extremities in multiple sclerosis: Case Series with 4- Year Follow-up. Archives of Physical Medicine and Rehabilitation. 2013;**94**(4):753-760

[95] Rensink M, et al. Task-oriented training in rehabilitation after stroke: systematic review. Journal of advanced nursing. 2009;**65**(4):737-754

[96] Almhdawi KA, et al. Efficacy of occupational therapy task-oriented approach in upper extremity post-stroke rehabilitation. Occupational therapy international. 2016;**23**(4):444-456

[97] Choi JU, Kang SH. The effects of patient-centered task-oriented training on balance activities of daily living and self-efficacy following stroke. Journal of physical therapy science. 2015;**27**(9):2985-2988

[98] Kim Y, Lee BH. Clinical usefulness of child-centered task-oriented training on balance ability in cerebral palsy. Journal of physical therapy science. 2013;**25**(8):947-951

[99] Test G, Test FR. The effects of a home-based task-oriented exercise programme on motor and balance performance in children with spastic cerebral palsy and severe traumatic brain injury. Journal of Motor Behavior. 2009;**42**(2):714-724

[100] Schneiberg S, et al. The effectiveness of task-oriented intervention and trunk restraint on upper limb movement quality in children with cerebral palsy. Developmental Medicine & Child Neurology. 2010;**52**(11):e245-e253

[101] Song C-S. Effects of task-oriented approach on affected arm function in children with spastic hemiplegia due to cerebral palsy. Journal of physical therapy science. 2014;**26**(6):797-800

[102] Moon J, Jung J, Hahm S. The effects of task-oriented training on hand dexterity and strength in children with spastic hemiplegic cerebral palsy: A preliminary study. The Journal of Physical Therapy Science. 2017;**29**(10):1800-1802

[103] Straudi S, Martinuzzi C, Pavarelli C, Charabati AS, Benedetti MG, Foti C, et al. A task-oriented circuit training in multiple sclerosis: A feasibility study. Elsevier, Science Direct. 2014;**37**(5-6):1-9

[104] Darwish MH, Shalaby NM, Ali AS. Effect of task oriented approach on balance in ataxic multiple sclerosis

patients. The medical journal of Cairo University. 2019;**87**(7):4789-4794

[105] Hassanin MA, Aly MG, Ahmed GM. Effect of task-oriented training on upper extremity function for patients with spinal cord and traumatic brain injuries: Systematic review. The Medical Journal of Cairo University. 2021;**89**(4):1731-1738

[106] Dennison A, Hirsch MA, Hammond FM. Rehabilitation with a mirror. Archives of Physical Medicine and Rehabilitation [Internet]. 2009;**90**(12):2155. Available from: http://www.archives-pmr.org/article/S000399930900759X/fulltext

[107] Lamont K, Chin M, Kogan M. Mirror box therapy – seeing is believing. Explorer. 2011;7(6):369-372

[108] Paik Y, Kim S, Lee J, Jeon B. Simple and task-oriented mirror therapy for upper extremity function in stroke patients: A pilot study. Hong Kong Journal of Occupational Therapy. 2014;**24**:6-12

[109] Lin KC, Chen YT, Huang PC, Wu CY, Huang WL, Yang HW, et al. Effect of mirror therapy combined with somatosensory stimulation on motor recovery and daily function in stroke patients: A pilot study. Journal of the Formosan Medical Association. 2014;**113**(7):422-428

[110] Michielsen ME, Selles RW, Van Der Geest JN, Eckhardt M, Yavuzer G, Stam HJ, et al. Motor recovery and cortical reorganization after mirror therapy in chronic stroke patients: A phase II randomized controlled trial. Neurorehabilitation and Neural Repair. 2011;**25**(3):223-233

[111] Dohle C, Püllen J, Nakaten A, Küst J, Rietz C, Karbe H. Mirror therapy promotes recovery from severe hemiparesis: A randomized controlled trial. Neurorehabilitation and Neural Repair. 2009;**23**(3):209-217

[112] Lin K, Chen Y, Huang P. Effect of mirror therapy combined with somatosensory stimulation on motor recovery and daily function in stroke patients: A pilot study. Journal of the Formosan Medical Association [Internet]. 2014;**113**(7):422-428. DOI: 10.1016/j.jfma.2012.08.008

[113] Golaszewski SM, Bergmann J, Christova M, Kunz AB, Kronbichler M, Rafolt D, et al. Modulation of motor cortex excitability by different levels of whole-hand afferent electrical stimulation. Clinical Neurophysiology. 2012;**123**(1):193-199

[114] Golaszewski SM, Bergmann J, Christova M, Nardone R, Kronbichler M, Rafolt D, et al. Increased motor cortical excitability after whole-hand electrical stimulation: A TMS study. Clinical Neurophysiology. 2010;**121**(2):248-254

[115] Chipchase LS, Schabrun SM, Hodges PW. Peripheral electrical stimulation to induce cortical plasticity: A systematic review of stimulus parameters. Clinical Neurophysiology. 2011;**122**(3):456-463

[116] Skubik-Peplaski CL. Environmental Influences on Occupational Therapy Practice uknowledge. 2012. p. 287

[117] De Luca R, Calabrò RS, Bramanti P. Cognitive rehabilitation after severe acquired brain injury: current evidence and future directions. Neuropsychological rehabilitation.2018;**28**(6):879-898

[118] Lee SW, Kielhofner G. Volition. Kielhofner's Model of Human Occupation. 2017:38-56

[119] Lin TT, Fisher G. Applying the model of human occupation during the pandemic stay-at-home order. Open J Occup Ther. 2020;**8**(4):1-7

[120] Strong S, Rigby P, Stewart D, Law M, Letts L, Cooper B. Application of the person-environment-occupation model: A practical tool. Canadian Journal of Occupational Therapy. 1999;**66**(3):122-133

[121] Black D. The Social Structure of Right and Wrong. United Kingdom: Academic Press; 2014. p. 169

[122] Wong AWK, Ng S, Dashner J, Baum MC, Hammel J, Magasi S, et al. Relationships between environmental factors and participation in adults with traumatic brain injury, stroke, and spinal cord injury: A cross-sectional multi-center study. Quality of Life Research. 2017;**26**(10):2633-2645

[123] Harrison M, Angarola R, Forsyth K, Irvine L. Defining the environment to support occupational therapy intervention in mental health practice. British Journal of Occupational Therapy. 2016;**79**(1):57-59

[124] Aybek S, Perez DL. Diagnosis and management of functional neurological disorder. BMJ. 2022;**376**:376

[125] Popkirov S, Stone J, Buchan AM. Functional neurological disorder. Stroke. 2020;**51**(5):1629-1635

[126] Hospital W. Standard of care. Functional neurologic disorder. The canadian journal of neurological sciences Inc. 2019;**48**:1-21

[127] Lehn A, Navaratnam D, Broughton M, Cheah V, Fenton A, Harm K, et al. Functional neurological disorders: effective teaching for health professionals. BMJ Neurology Open. 28 Jun 2020;**2**(1):000065

[128] Foundation W, Press JH, Practice C. Neurological rehabilitation. HHS Public Access. 2020;**75**(9):1132-1141

[129] Stone J. Functional neurological disorders: The neurological assessment as treatment. BMJ Journals. 2016;**16**(1):7-17

[130] Vassilopoulos A, Mohammad S, Dure L, Kozlowska K, Fobian AD. Treatment approaches for functional neurological disorders in children. Curr Treat Options Neurol [Internet]. 2022;**24**(2):77-97. DOI: 10.1007/s11940-022-00708-5

[131] Glass A, Zazulia AR. Clinical skills: Neurological examination. 2011. Available from: https://neurology.wustl.edu/wp-content/uploads/2022/06/Neurological-Exam-Lecture-Notes.pdf

[132] Lima VLCC. Neurofunctional speech rehabilitation in cerebral palsy: A study on the combination of transcranial direct current stimulation and an integrative speech therapy program. Austin Journal of Clinical Neurology. 2017;**4**(4):1113

[133] Langhorne P, Bernhardt J, Kwakkel G. Stroke rehabilitation. Lancet. 2011;**377**(9778):1693-1702

[134] Edmans J. Occupational therapy and stroke. Wiley Online library. Blackwell Publishing Ltd.; 2010. DOI: 10.1002/9781444323801

[135] Officer A, Groce NE. Key concepts in disability. Lancet. London, England. 2009;**374**(9704):1795-1796

[136] Barbey A, Pjanic I, Studer H, Bischoff N, Bassetti CLA, Aybek S. Management of functional neurological disorders (FND): Experience from a Swiss FND Clinic. Clinical and Translational Neuroscience. 2022;**6**(1):2

[137] Brewer L, Horgan F, Hickey A, Williams D. Stroke rehabilitation: Recent advances and future therapies. QJM. 2013;**106**(1):11-25

Chapter 7

Nutritional Support in Stroke Neurorehabilitation

Andrés J. Ursa Herguedas and Emilio J. Guzón González

Abstract

Acquired brain injury (ABI) due to stroke or cerebrovascular accident (CVA) is a frequent pathology that leaves sequelae, produces great personal and family suffering and has a great economic impact on health systems. Translational research and clinical evidence have revealed the existence of an intestinal dysbiosis in these patients before and after stroke that, ultimately, through the microbiota-gut-brain axis, is capable of producing neuroinflammation, negatively impacting the evolution of stroke and delaying functional recovery in the neurorehabilitation process. Individualized dietary intervention is proposed in order to reverse intestinal dysbiosis until reaching eubiosis and facilitate recovery. For this it would be necessary to have the figure of the nutritionist-dietician in the multidisciplinary team. The objective of this chapter is to report on the importance of nutritional intervention in stroke to obtain better results. Research in this regard must continue as several questions remain unanswered.

Keywords: stroke, cerebrovascular accident, gut microbiota, gut dysbiosis, microbiota-gut-brain axis, neuroinflammation

1. Introduction

Stroke or cerebrovascular accident (CVA) is one of the most frequent reasons for urgent neurological care, it is one of the main causes of death and disability in adults and it entails an enormous human and economic cost in developed countries. In recent decades, various advances have been made in the treatment of stroke, such as early medical-surgical care, the creation of stroke units in health centers and rehabilitation treatment. Neurorehabilitation, applied in the different evolutionary stages of stroke, is one of the most decisive interventions when it comes to addressing neurological injuries and their functional repercussions of stroke [1]. Ischemic stroke is responsible for most cerebrovascular accidents, with hemorrhagic stroke being the second most frequent. The annual incidence of stroke in Spain is 156 new cases per 100,000 inhabitants and its prevalence is 500–600 cases per 100,000 inhabitants [2].

Occlusion of the middle cerebral artery produces ischemia in the affected territory, followed by an inflammatory and immune response [3]. Neurological deficits are usually present from the first moment.

 IntechOpen

In various studies on the gut microbiota (GM) in stroke patients, the presence of dysbiosis, altered intestinal permeability, the passage of bacterial lipopolysaccharides through the intestinal barrier into the bloodstream, the maintenance of a systemic low-grade inflammatory state (SLGIS) and neuroinflammation [4].

Given this state of knowledge, we have to find out what is the degree of contribution of SLGIS and neuroinflammation to the establishment of stroke? Can nutritional intervention to achieve intestinal eubiosis contribute to improving stroke prognosis and/or better functional recovery? Translational research and clinical evidence offer us the opportunity to systematically intervene in the stroke neurorehabilitation process with nutritional support in order to reverse the inflammatory state and facilitate the recovery process. To achieve this goal, it would be necessary to include a nutritionist-dietician in the multidisciplinary team that cares for these patients. We cannot forget the application of a holistic approach to the entire neurorehabilitation process, based on clinical and scientific evidence, all within the context of integrative medicine.

2. Reciprocal influence between microbiota, gut and brain

The intestine and the brain are in constant communication and for this they use different pathways such as endocrine, nervous and immune signaling. The balance between the different symbiotic bacterial species that populate the GM contributes to homeostasis through its participation in various metabolic pathways, the supply of nutrients such as vitamins and short-chain fatty acids (SCFA), stimulating the immune system, facilitating metabolism of substances not digestible by the host, acting on the metabolism of drugs and other xenobiotics, while avoiding colonization by pathogenic species [5].

This exchange of information occurs both via the nerves via neurotransmitters and via the blood (hormones, cytokines, metabolites ...). The central nervous system (CNS), the autonomic nervous system (ANS), the enteric nervous system (ENS), the neuroendocrine and neuroimmune systems contribute to this process, forming a fluid exchange network [6, 7].

In murine models, it has been proven that, by stimulating the afferent pathways of the vagus nerve, through the production of metabolites (neurotransmitters, hormones, SCFA) or through interactions with the immune system, GM is capable of modulating brain activity. Similarly, signals are emitted from the CNS that affect the MI [8].

An important pathway by which gut microbes and their metabolites communicate with the CNS involves the cells that make up the gut endocrine system [9]. This communication is mediated by several microbially derived molecules including SCFA, secondary bile acids, and tryptophan metabolites [10]. SCFAs have been implicated as the main signaling molecules that mediate host-microbe communication through enteroendocrine cells (EECs) and enterochromaffin cells (ECCs). SCFAs are generated by the microbial fermentation of resistant starch and non-starch polysaccharides that reach the intestine. These molecules play a role in host energy computation, as well as other functions such as stimulation of local blood flow, fluid and electrolyte absorption, and intestinal mucosal proliferation [11].

SCFAs propagate signals primarily through interaction with EECs, ECCs, and the mucosal immune system. Some cross the intestinal barrier, enter the systemic circulation, and can cross the blood-brain barrier [12]. It has been shown that SCFA production stimulates L cells located in the distal ileum to secrete peptide YY and glucagon-like peptide-1 (GLP-1), which induce satiety and behavioral changes [13]. Among other SCFAs, acetate, butyrate, and propionate modulate GLP-1 expression and secretion via free fatty acid receptor 2 (FFAR2)/G protein-coupled receptor 43 (GPR43) and FFAR3/GPR41 in L cells [13]. Vagal receptors detect gut regulatory peptides, inflammatory molecules, dietary components, and bacterial metabolites and send this information to the CNS [14].

The blood-brain barrier (BBB) regulates the transit of molecules between the circulatory system and the cerebrospinal fluid of the CNS. In murine models, GM can regulate the expression of intestinal cell-to-cell tight junction proteins, including occludin and claudin-5, allowing BBB permeability to be reduced [15]. Systemic immune activation can cause disruptive changes in the BBB and is often modeled using lipopolysaccharides (LPS). Studies evaluating the effects of LPS in vivo on BBB function only showed disruption 60% of the time [16].

3. Relationship between intestinal dysbiosis and neuropsychiatric pathology

The presence of intestinal dysbiosis can affect the proper functioning of the body and is associated with the development of digestive pathologies, as well as other apparatus and systems such as the immune, metabolic, cardiocirculatory or nervous. In recent years, numerous studies have found links between GM alterations and the most frequent neuropsychiatric disorders such as depression, Alzheimer's disease, Parkinson's disease, autism spectrum disorder, psychosis and demyelinating pathology such as multiple sclerosis [17, 18]. It has been shown that nearly 90% of stroke cases may be related to behavioral factors including poor diet, smoking, and low physical activity, as well as obesity, hypertension, and/or diabetes mellitus. Several studies consider GM as a risk factor for stroke [19].

Under normal conditions, commensal microbes inhabit the outer layer of the colon. The mucus that covers it, rich in glycoproteins, is a source of energy for the microbiota when the amount of fiber in the diet is not sufficient. This circumstance favors the possibility of colonization by pathogenic microorganisms [20]. The inner layer is generally free of bacteria and serves to protect epithelial cells from microbial contact through physical separation and innate immune mechanisms including antimicrobial peptides and adaptive immune mechanisms such as secretory IgA [21].

In murine models it has been shown that stress can cause alterations in the intestinal barrier by directly modulating epithelial permeability and by altering the properties of the intestinal mucosal layer. This fact produces a greater translocation of intestinal microbes or molecules associated with microbes [22]. In these models, it has been shown that the permeability of the jejunum and colon increases in response to either acute or chronic stress [23]. Bacteria, such as Escherichia coli, and their products, as well as bacterial LPS, lead to a pro-inflammatory environment in the gut. Stress-induced changes in the expression of messenger RNA encoding tight junction proteins have also been described in the colon and jejunum [24]. In addition, stress leads to a less protective mucus layer through catecholamine signaling, which alters the composition and size of secreted mucus, as the ANS modulates mucus secretion by intestinal goblet cells, thereby affecting the thickness and quality of the intestinal mucus layer [25].

It is possible that the changes in GM composition observed in murine models of brain injury are the result of altered mucoprotein production and goblet cell population size mediated by increased sympathetic nervous system signaling [26]. Furthermore, epinephrine and norepinephrine have been shown to increase the virulence properties of various enteric pathogens as well as non-pathogenic microbes through stimulation of natural immune sensing mechanisms [27]. Substantial roles for gut microbial regulation of autoimmunity, inflammation, and immune cell trafficking have been identified in mouse models of multiple sclerosis and stroke [28, 29]. Toll-like receptors 3 and 7 recognize viral RNA, and Toll-like receptors 2 and 4 recognize peptidoglycan and LPS. These receptors are expressed in both the murine and human ENS [30].

Under normal conditions, various types of microorganisms and macromolecules manage to cross the intestinal barrier through the M cells, which are part of the lymphoid tissue associated with the intestinal mucosa. This activity allows the constant checking of microorganisms and various molecules [31]. On the other hand, Paneth cells detect bacteria autonomously through the activation of the Toll-like receptor dependent on the MyD88 gene, responsible for the innate immune response to pathogens, which triggers antimicrobial factors and, ultimately, limits the penetration bacteria in host tissue [32]. Microbes and microbial-derived ligands help maintain the tight junctions between cells that are critical for the integrity of the intestinal barrier [33]. All these mechanisms and their alteration for different reasons, make it possible for information to reach the CNS and various types of reactions to occur, such as neuroinflammation and accelerate brain aging, contribute to the genesis of various neuropsychiatric diseases and hinder or delay recovery of ABI.

4. Neuroinflammation in the context of stroke

Increasing evidence suggests that intestinal inflammation together with the immune response plays an essential role in the pathophysiology of stroke and this may become an important therapeutic target for the treatment of ABI [34]. The different communication pathways between the microbiota, intestine and brain, the increase in intestinal permeability and the passage of molecules through the BBB would make it possible to activate the immune cells of the CNS [35].

The BBB is made up of blood vessels that allow substances to pass into the CNS in a very selective manner to maintain correct homeostasis, guaranteeing correct neural function. The properties of this barrier are due to its architecture and the cells that make it up, the most important being the endothelial cells (EC), which have a great capacity to very selectively regulate the movement of ions, molecules and cells between the blood and the brain. Specific transporters are expressed in these cells that allow a selective passage of substances in both directions. To limit passage of immune cells into the CNS, ECs express very few leukocyte adhesion molecules. The set of all these properties allows the maintenance of cerebral homeostasis in a healthy situation [36].

The inflammatory process during cerebral ischemia involves the participation of glia and microglia, mediating the migration, infiltration, and accumulation of leukocytes to the brain parenchyma during ischemia. In ABI, the expression of cytokines (IL-1β, TNFα, IFNγ) and chemokines such as CCL2 (MCP-1), CCL5 (RANTES) and CXCL1 (GRO-α) has been demonstrated, which precedes the infiltration of leukocytes towards ischemic injury, acting through its receptors CCR2, CCR5 and CXCR2, respectively. Inflammation contributes to tissue injury during the early phase of the hypoxic-ischemic response and during the healing process in the late phase of cerebral ischemia. Thus, chemokines exert an inflammatory action against brain damage, although some of them have a neuroprotective effect by inducing the synthesis of growth factors that contribute to brain regeneration based on neuroplasticity, all if the attention process of the patient is carried out in the optimal time and circumstances [37].

The changes in GM in patients who have suffered a stroke have been documented in several studies [38], but it is in murine models that the sequence of events and the repercussions for the evolution and functional recovery of the stroke have been appreciated. In murine models using two types of acute middle cerebral artery occlusion, large stroke lesions were found to cause intestinal dysbiosis, which in turn affected stroke outcome through immune-mediated mechanisms. Reduced species diversity and bacterial overgrowth of Bacteroidetes were identified as hallmarks of post-stroke dysbiosis, which was associated with intestinal barrier dysfunction and reduced intestinal motility following injury progression. The impact of the microbiota on immunity and stroke outcome was transmissible by microbiota transplantation [39].

5. Nutritional intervention in stroke

The composition of GM is defined by many factors, including the way of being born, the consumption of antibiotics, infection processes, stress, customs, ethnicity, habitat, hygienic habits, genetics and diet among others. Although used infrequently as an intervention specifically targeting GM, diet can have profound, rapid, and reproducible effects on GM structure in humans and animals [40]. Clinical experience and published studies, both in humans and in murine models, invite us to implement the analysis of GM in patients who have suffered a stroke and, in the case of intestinal dysbiosis, to intervene with the modification of the diet until eubiosis is acquired. At this level, there are still some doubts such as the optimal time to start the dietary intervention to act on dysbiosis, that is, in what phase of the stroke would it start? **Table 1** shows the stroke phases, their approximate duration and the units where they are treated according to Murie-Fernández et al. [1].

If we are willing to intervene in stroke patients, it would be convenient to add the figure of the nutritionist-dietician in the team that cares for stroke patients. **Table 2** shows the members of the multidisciplinary team in stroke rehabilitation according to Murie-Fernández et al. [1], to which we include the figure of the degree in human nutrition and dietetics.

A diet adapted to each patient who has suffered a stroke with intestinal dysbiosis, with adequate dietary fiber, the administration of probiotics, symbiotic, etc., could contribute to a better evolution and functional recovery to the current on

Phase	Duration	Unit of stay
Acute	2–3 months	Hospitalization
Subacute	6 to 18 months	Rehabilitation, day hospital
Chronic	From 24 months	Residency, physiotherapy

Table 1.
Phases of stroke, duration and where it is treated according to Murie-Fernández et al. [1].

Discipline	Function	Intervenes in phase
Neurology	Diagnostic	Acute
Nursing	Acute hospitalization care	Acute
Neurosurgery	Clot removal (if applicable)	Acute
Nutrition and dietetics	Diet planning according to the patient's evolution	?
Physical medicine and rehabilitation	Treatment protocol	Acute/subacute
Physiotherapist	Techniques, treatments and strategies to recover damaged functions	Subacute
Neuropsychologist	Action on behavior, emotions, etc	Acute/subacute
Speech therapy	Acting on dysphagia, dysphonia, dysarthria, aphasia, etc	Subacute
Occupational therapy	Stimulation, reeducation,...	Subacute
Orthopedic technician	Adaptations	Subacute/chronic
Social work	Comprehensive management	Subacute

Table 2.
Multidisciplinary team in stroke rehabilitation according to Murie-Fernández et al. [1] and completed by A. Ursa and E. Guzón.

neuroinflammation [41, 42]. More studies are still needed to expand knowledge, clear up doubts and design protocols adaptable to different patients and contexts.

6. Conclusions

Acute brain injuries such as stroke induce gut dysbiosis and, in turn, changes in GM influence neuroinflammation and thus function in ABI. GM is a key regulator in preparing the neuroinflammatory response to brain injury. These findings highlight the role that GM plays as a therapeutic target to protect brain function after acute brain injury. Dietary intervention in patients with stroke, either by nasogastric tube in case of unconsciousness or orally if there is no alteration of consciousness, would contribute to a better evolution of the stroke and functional recovery. Much remains to be discovered about the specific mechanisms by which GM is involved in the gut-brain axis and in disease development. Current evidence encourages us to continue researching on this topic.

Funding

This chapter has been funded by the Institute of Integrative Medicine (Valladolid, Spain).

Conflict of interest

There is no conflict of interest.

Abbreviations

CVA	cerebrovascular accident
ABI	acquired brain damage injury
GM	gut microbiota
SLGIS	systemic low-grade inflammatory state
SCFA	short chain fatty acids
CNS	central nervous system
ANS	autonomic nervous system
ENS	enteric nervous system
EEC	enteroendocrine cells
ECC	enterochromaffin cells
GLP-1	glucagon-like peptide 1
FFAR2/3	free fatty acid receptor 2/3
GPR 43/41	G43/41 protein-coupled receptor
BBB	blood-brain barrier
LPS	lipopolysaccharides
EC	endothelial cells

Author details

Andrés J. Ursa Herguedas[1,2,3,4,5]* and Emilio J. Guzón González[6,7,8,9,10,11,12]*

1 Institute of Integrative Medicine, Valladolid, Spain

2 Medicine and Surgery, Complutense University of Madrid, Spain

3 Junta de Castilla y León, Valladolid, Spain

4 Rehabilitation and Pain, University of Valladolid, Spain

5 Clinical Neurophysiology, University of Valladolid, Spain

6 Human Nutrition and Dietetics, University of Valladolid, Spain

7 Food Science and Technology, Complutense University of Madrid, Spain

8 Clinical and Community Nutrition, University of Alicante, Spain

9 Public Health, Carlos III Health Institute in Madrid, Spain

10 Health Sciences, Doctoral School of the University of Valladolid, Spain

11 Food and Nutrition Research Team (ALINUT), University of Alicante, Spain

12 Miguel de Cervantes European University, Valladolid, Spain

*Address all correspondence to: ajursa@educa.jcyl.es and guzonemilio@gmail.com

IntechOpen

© 2022 The Author(s). Licensee IntechOpen. This chapter is distributed under the terms of the Creative Commons Attribution License (http://creativecommons.org/licenses/by/3.0), which permits unrestricted use, distribution, and reproduction in any medium, provided the original work is properly cited.

References

[1] Murie-Fernández M, Irimia P, Martínez-Vila E, John MM, Teasell R. Neurorehabilitation after stroke. Neurology. 2010;**25**(3):189-196. DOI: 10.1016/S0213-4853(10)70008-6

[2] Soler Suñer R et al. Treatise on Neurological Nursing the Person, the Disease and Care. 3rd ed. Spain: Spanish Society of Neurological Nursing (SEDENE); 2013

[3] Hossmann KA. Pathophysiology and therapy of experimental stroke. Cellular and Molecular Neurobiology. 2006;**26**(7-8):1057-1083. DOI: 10.1007/s10571-006-9008-1

[4] Li N, Wang X, Sun C, Xinwei W, Mei L, Si Y, et al. Change of intestinal microbiota in cerebral ischemic stroke patients. BMC Microbiology. 2019;**19**:191. DOI: 10.1186/s12866-019-1552-1

[5] Martin CR, Osadchiy V, Kalani A, Mayer EA. The brain-gut-microbiome Axis. Cellular and Molecular Gastroenterology and Hepatology. 2018;**6**(2):133-148. DOI: 10.1016/j.jcmgh.2018.04.003

[6] Gómez-Eguílaz M, Ramón-Trapero JL, Pérez-Martínez L, Blanco JR. The microbiota-gut-brain axis and its large projections. Neurology. 2019;**68**(3):111-117

[7] Muller PA, Schneeberger M, Matheis F, et al. Microbiota modulate sympathetic neurons via a gut–brain circuit. Nature. 2020;**583**:441-446. DOI: 10.1038/s41586-020-2474-7

[8] Bravo JA, Forsythe P, Chew MV, Escaravage E, Savignac HM, Dinan TG, et al. Lactobacillus strain ingestion regulates emotional behavior and central GABA receptor expression in a mouse via nerve vague. Proceedings of the National Academy Science USA. 2011;**108**:16050-16055. DOI: 10.1073/pnas.1102999108

[9] Furness JB, Rivera LR, Cho HJ, Bravo DM, Callaghan B. The gut as a sensory organ. Nature Reviews: Gastroenterology & Hepatology. 2013;**10**:729-740. DOI: 10.1038/nrgastro.2013.180

[10] Yano JM, Yu K, Donaldson GP, Shastri GG, Ann P, Ma L, et al. Indigenous bacteria of the gut microbiota regulate host serotonin biosynthesis. Cell. 2015;**161**:264-276. DOI: 10.1016/j.cell.2015.02.047

[11] Topping DE, Clifton PM. Short-chain fatty acids and human colonic function: Roles of starch-resistant and non-starch polysaccharides. Physiological Reviews. 2001;**81**:1031-1064. DOI: 10.1152/physrev.2001.81.3.1031

[12] Haghikia A, Jorg S, Duscha A, Berg J, Manzel A, Waschbisch A, et al. Dietary fatty acids have a direct impact on autoimmunity from the central nervous system through the small intestine. Immunity. 2015;**43**:817-829. DOI: 10.1016/j.immune.2015.09.007

[13] Tolhurst G, Heffron H, Lam YS, Parker HE, Habib AM, Diakogiannaki E, et al. Short-chain fatty acids stimulate glucagon-like peptide 1 secretion through the G protein-coupled receptor FFAR2. Diabetes. 2012;**61**:364-371. DOI: 10.2337/db11-1019

[14] de Lartigue G, de La Serre CB, Raybould HE. Vagal afferent neurons in high-fat diet-induced obesity; intestinal microflora, intestinal inflammation and cholecystokinin. Physiological behavior.

2011;**105**:100-105. DOI: 10.1016/j.physbeh.2011.02.040

[15] Braniste V, Al-Asmakh M, Kowal C, Anuar F, Abbaspour A, Toth M, et al. Gut microbiota influences blood-brain barrier permeability in mice. Science Translational Medicine. 2014;**6**:263ra158

[16] Varatharaj A, Galea I. The blood-brain barrier in systemic inflammation. Brain, Behavior, and Immunity. 2017;**60**:1-12. DOI: 10.1016/j.bbi.2016.03.010

[17] Codagnone MG, Spichak S, O'Mahony SM, O'Leary OF, Clarke G, Stanton C, et al. Programming bugs: Microbiota and the developmental origins of brain health and disease. Biological Psychiatry. 2019;**85**:150-163. DOI: 10.1016/j.biopsych.2018.06.014

[18] Grochwska M, Laskus T, Radkowski M. Gut microbiota in neurological disorders. Archivum Immunologiae et Therapiae Experimentalis. 2019;**67**:375-383. DOI: 10.1007/s00005-019-00561-6

[19] Zeng X, Gao X, Peng Y, Wu Q, Zhu J, Tan C, et al. An increased risk of stroke correlates with a higher burden of opportunistic pathogens and reduced levels of butyrate-producing bacteria in the gut. Frontiers in Cellular and Infection Microbiology. 2019;**9**:4. DOI: 10.3389/fcimb.2019.00004

[20] Desai MS, Seekatz AM, Koropatkin NM, Kamada N, Hickey CA, Wolter M, et al. A gut microbiota deprived of dietary fiber degrades the mucosal barrier of the colon and increases susceptibility to pathogens. Cell. 2016;**167**:1339-1353

[21] Johansson ME, Larsson JM, Hansson GC. The two mucus layers of the colon are organized by the mucin MUC2, while the outer layer is a legislator of host-microbial interactions. Proceedings of the National Academy Science USA. 2011;**108**(Supplement 1): 4659-4665. DOI: 10.1073/pnas.1006451107

[22] Santos J, Yang PC, Soderholm JD, Benjamin M, Perdue MH. Role of mast cells in chronic stress-induced colonic epithelial barrier dysfunction in the rat. Intestine. 2001;**48**:630-636. DOI: 10.1136/gut.48.5.630

[23] Saunders PR, Santos J, Hanssen NP, Yates D, Groot JA, Perdue MH. Physical and psychological stress in rats enhances colonic epithelial permeability through peripheral CRH. Digestive Diseases and Sciences. 2002;**47**:208-215. DOI: 10.1023/a:1013204612762

[24] Lauffer A, Vanuytsel T, Vanormelingen C, Vanheel H, Salim Rasoel S, Toth J, et al. Subacute stress and chronic stress interact to decrease gut barrier function in rat. Stress. 2016;**19**:225-234. DOI: 10.3109/10253890.2016.1154527

[25] Da Silva S, Robbe-Masselot C, Ait-Belgnaoui A, Mancuso A, Mercade-Loubiere M, Salvador-Cartier C, et al. Stress interrupts the intestinal mucosal barrier in rats through the change of O-glycosylation of mucin: Prevention by probiotic treatment. American Journal of Physiology. Gastrointestinal and Liver Physiology. 2014;**307**:G420-G429. DOI: 10.1152/ajpgi.00290.2013

[26] Houlden A, Goldrick M, Brough D, Vizi ES, Lenart N, Martinez B, et al. Brain injury induces specific changes in the cecal microbiota of mice through altered autonomic activity and mucoprotein production. Brain, Behavior, and Immunity. 2016;**57**:10-20. DOI: 10.1016/j.bbi.2016.04.003

[27] Hughes DT, Sperandio V. Cross-kingdom signaling: Communication between bacteria and their hosts. Nature Reviews. Microbiology. 2008;**6**:111-120. DOI: 10.1038/nrmicro1836

[28] Wang Y, Telesford KM, Ochoa-Reparaz J, Haque-Begum S, Christy M, Kasper EJ, et al. An intestinal commensal symbiosis factor controls neuroinflammation through TLR2-mediated CD39 signaling. Common Naturals. 2014;**5**:4432. DOI: org/10.1038/ncomms5432

[29] Benakis C, Brea D, Caballero S, Faraco G, Moore J, Murphy M, et al. Commensal microbiota affects ischemic stroke outcome by regulating T cells intestinal gamma delta. Nature Medicine. 2016;**22**:516-523. DOI: 10.1038/nm.4068

[30] Brun P, Giron MC, Qesari PA, Caputi V, Zoppellaro C, et al. Toll-like receptor 2 regulates intestinal inflammation by controlling the integrity of the enteric nervous system. Gastroenterology. 2013;**145**:1323-1333

[31] Kucharzik T, Lugering N, Rautenberg K, Lugering A, Schmidt MA, Stoll R, et al. Role of M cells in intestinal barrier function. Annals New York Academic Science. 2000;**915**:171-183. DOI: 10.1111/j.1749-6632.2000.tb05240.x

[32] Vaishnava S, Behrendt CL, Ismail AS, Eckmann L, Hooper LV. Paneth cells directly sense intestinal commensals and maintain homeostasis at the intestinal host microbial interface. Proceedings of the National Academy Science USA. 2008;**105**:20858-20863. DOI: 10.1073/pnas.0808723105

[33] Rakoff-Nahoum S, Paglino J, Eslami-Varzaneh F, Edberg S, Medzhitov R. Recognition of commensal microflora by toll-like receptors is required for intestinal homeostasis. Cell. 2004;**118**:229-241. DOI: 10.1016/j.cell.2004.07.002

[34] Iadecola C, Anrather J. The immunology of stroke: From mechanisms to translation. Nature Medicine. 2011;**17**(7):796-808. DOI: 10.1038/nm.2399

[35] Erny D, Hrabe de Angelis AL, Jaitin D, Wieghofer P, Staszewski O, David E, et al. The host microbiota constantly controls microglia maturation and function in the CNS. Nature Neuroscience. 2015;**18**:965-977

[36] Daneman R, Prat A. The blood–brain barrier. Cold Spring Harbor Perspectives in Biology. 2015;**7**(1):a020412. DOI: 10.1101/cshperspect.a020412

[37] Blanco-Álvarez VM, Soto-Rodríguez G, González-Barrios J, Beltrán-Galindo O, Martínez-Fong D. Neuroinflammatory and neurotrophic action of chemokines during a cerebral ischemic process. Revista de Especialidades Medico Quirurgicas. 2015;**20**:184-192

[38] Li N, Wang X, Sun C, Wu X, Lu M, Si Y, et al. Gut microbiota change in patients with cerebral ischemic stroke. Microbiology BMC. 2019;**19**(1):1-8. DOI: 10.1186/s12866-019-1552-1

[39] Singh V, Roth S, Llovera G, Sadler R, Garzetti D, Stecher B, et al. Microbiota dysbiosis controls the neuroinflammatory response after stroke. The Journal of Neuroscience. 2016;**36**(28):7428-7440. DOI: 10.1523/JNEUROSCI.1114-16.2016

[40] David LA, Maurice CF, Carmody RN, Gootenberg DB, Button JE, Wolfe BE, et al. Diet rapidly and reproducibly alters the human gut microbiome. Nature. 2014;**505**:559-563. DOI: 10.1038/nature12820

[41] Sanz Paris A, Álvarez Ballano D, de Diego GP, Lofablos Callau F, Albero GR. Cerebrovascular accident: Nutrition as a pathogenic and preventive factor. Post stroke nutritional support. Hospital Nutrition. 2009;**2**(2):38-55

[42] Bretón I, Cuerda C, Camblor M, Velasco C, Frías L, Higuera I, et al. Nutrition in stroke patients. Hospital Nutrition. 2013;**6**(1):39-48

Chapter 8

Mild Cognitive Impairment: An Overview

Biraj Bhattarai and Hema Nagaraj

Abstract

Heterogeneity of symptoms within and among mild cognitive impairment (MCI) individuals often makes it challenging to document cases clinically. Number of diagnostic criteria have been proposed in recent decades. MOCA and MMSE are two tests useful for the assessment of MCI, besides the neuroimaging studies with MRI and PET scan, have provided promising results in the early diagnosis of MCI. Lifestyle changes and cognitive training have been found to be more effective in the treatment of individuals with MCI.

Keywords: cognitive impairment, amnestic, non-amnestic, MoCA, MMSE, cognitive training

1. Introduction

1.1 Cognitive decline in aging

Changes in brain morphology resulting from normal aging have been documented in neuroimaging studies. The results show that there are alterations in white matter integrity, white matter hyper-intensities, and reduced hippocampal volumes [1–3].

Cognitive decline is a common phenomenon associated with normal aging and is getting a lot of attention among clinicians. Some of the earlier labels such as "benign senescent forgetfulness," [4] "age-associated memory impairment" (AAMI) [5], "age-associated cognitive decline" (AACD) [6], and "age-related cognitive decline" [7] are frequently used to describe the deterioration in cognition.

The decline in cognitive performance with aging is due to several cognitive processes, including a reduction in processing speed, working memory capacity, and loss of sensory input. This thereby results in deficits in encoding, storing, and retrieving information, but cognitive capability remains unaffected [8, 9]. The problems are mainly noted while retrieving information from the long-term and short-term memory store, where the retrieval of information is slower in the former, and the amount of information that can be stored decreases in the latter [9].

During the aging process, the onset of dementia has been widely reported. Recently, the label "mild cognitive impairment (MCI)" has been used to signify the intermediate condition between dementia and normal aging [10]. Cases presenting with the following signs and symptoms such as (i) informant-corroborated history of memory symptoms, (ii) impairment in memory when measured objectively (usually <1.5 standard deviations on a verbal memory test), (iii) spared general cognition, (iv) activities of daily living (ADL) well preserved, and (v) no dementia are recommended to use this label [11]. Recent criteria proposed include the following cognitive domains for diagnosing MCI, and four subgroups made are of (1) only memory deficit; (2) memory deficit along with deficits in other cognitive domains; (3) deficit in the non-memory domain; and (4) non-memory domain deficit along with deficits in other cognitive domains [12, 13]. Evidence suggests that cognitive decline in MCI has no adverse effects on the activities of daily living in contrast to dementia, and this is consistent with the definition of "mild neurocognitive decline"(NCD) from DSM-V [14]. Cognitive decline was studied in individuals with Alzheimer's disease (AD), mild cognitive impairment (MCI), and normal cognition for 11 years, and it was concluded that the cognitive capacity in the normal group declined at a slower extent than in the MCI group and that of the MCI group declined at slower extent than the group with Alzheimer's disease [15]. Studies report that all cases diagnosed as MCI do not progress to dementia [12, 13].

There is substantial evidence that neuropathological alterations occur several years before the clinical manifestation of Alzheimer's disease (AD) [16, 17] and that subtle cognitive abnormalities persist up to 9 years before a dementia diagnosis [18].

As a result of these findings, researchers have coined the term moderate cognitive impairment (MCI), which was coined by Flicker, Ferris, and Reisberg [19]. MCI is defined by Petersen and colleagues [16] as a transitional, preclinical state characterized by intermediate symptomatology between cognitive changes associated with healthy aging and the more pathological alterations associated with Alzheimer's disease [20].

Memory complaints (confirmed by an informant), objective evidence of memory impairment (for age and education level), generally intact overall cognitive function, essentially preserved activities of daily living, and the absence of dementia are all clinical criteria for diagnosing MCI, according to the American Academy of Neurology [21]. Separate subgroups of MCI have been found more recently [12] based on the element of cognition that is most impacted. Memory loss is the most significant symptom of amnestic MCI (a-MCI). In longitudinal studies, this kind of MCI is the most frequent and is most likely to be related to conversion to AD.

Figure 1 depicts current perspectives on the shift from healthy cognitive aging to amnestic MCI and Alzheimer's disease. Single non-memory domain MCI (sd-MCI) is another subtype of MCI that is characterized by significant abnormalities in linguistic skills, executive function, or visuospatial function [12]. Finally, multiple domain MCI (MD-MCI) is characterized by the involvement of multiple cognitive domains and can occur with or without memory problems (MD-MCI + a). According to epidemiologic research, persons diagnosed with MCI are substantially more likely to develop AD or dementia within 5 years than those without MCI. In one study, 56% of amnestic MCI individuals and 50% of non-amnestic MCI participants transitioned to Alzheimer's disease or dementia within 4 years [22].

Table 1 summarizes the four widely recognized subtypes of MCI. Generally, a case of MCI is classified in one of the following four subtypes as per four essential characteristics, (1) Complaints of cognitive problems; (2) Memory impairment; (3) Impaired or spared functional ability, and (4) Presence or absence of dementia. Within MCI, amnestic versus non-amnestic MCI is classified based on memory impairment. Suppose an individual is objectively confirmed to have memory-related issues. In that case, it is classified within amnestic types, and if s/he has issues related to other domains of cognition rather than memory, then it is confirmed to be

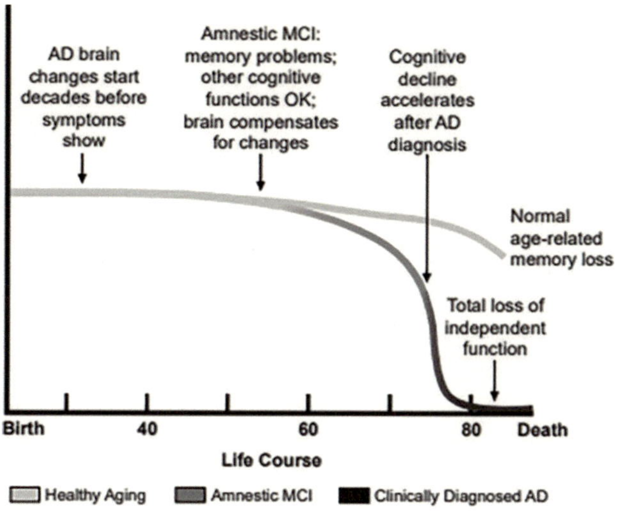

Figure 1.
Current perspectives on the shift from healthy cognitive aging to amnestic MCI and Alzheimer's disease.

Subtypes	Characteristics
Amnestic MCI (Single Domain)	•Subjective or proxy cognitive complaint •Objective memory impairment •Relatively intact functional ability •Not demented
Amnestic MCI (Multiple Domain)	•Subjective or proxy cognitive complaint •Objective impairment in memory and at least one other cognitive domain •Relatively intact functional ability •Not demented
Non-Amnestic MCI (Single Domain)	•Subjective or proxy cognitive complaint •Objective impairment in one non-memory domain •Relatively intact functional ability •Not demented
Non-Amnestic MCI (Multiple Domain)	•Personal or proxy cognitive complaint •Objective impairment in two or more non-memory domains •Relatively Intact functional ability •Not demented

Table 1.
Four widely recognized subtypes of mild cognitive impairment (MCI).

non-amnestic. Further, if a single aspect of cognitive function is affected, it is termed a single domain, and if two or more elements are involved, it is confirmed to be multiple domains.

1.2 MCI—signs and symptoms

There are three main types of trajectories seen in cognitive decline, which are (1) Stable pattern, observed for the impaired language skills; (2) Gradual pattern, noted for immediate recall, inhibition, and visuospatial skills; (3) Stable period followed by accelerated decline pattern, seen in delayed recall, visuospatial memory, and working memory skill [23]. It has been reported that episodic and working memory are the domains that are affected to a greater extent among MCI individuals and present with the fastest decline in those individuals who progress to other groups like dementia. These studies have consistently found that memory deficits are the major deficits reported by individuals with MCI or their caregivers [24].

Individuals with MCI exhibit a wide range of difficulties in multiple areas of cognitive functioning, such as attention, memory (primary and secondary), visuospatial ability, and language and executive functioning [6]. MCI has been considered a "syndrome" due to the presence of a cluster of symptoms centered around major neuropsychological manifestations, such as (i) complaints of noticeable cognitive decline, (ii) memory deficit observable on tests, and (iii) spared activities of daily living except mild deficit in instrumental activities of daily living [25, 26]. Evidence suggests individual with MCI usually presents with the complaint of a certain decline in normal cognitive functioning. Evidence shows that mood variations are a good predictor of MCI [26–28]. An important diagnostic variable is the presence of preserved activities of daily living. However, it is observed that the instrumental activities of daily living are much more affected than the ADLs [26]. For example, an auto-driver with MCI might face more difficulty executing his skill/or job effectively.

Regarding the diagnosis of MCI, there is a considerable amount of debate going on. Previous literature has reported that the condition of MCI is characterized solely by memory impairment. Further studies, however, supported that MCI could be an impairment in the non-memory domain alone or a condition with multiple cognitive components (executive function, memory, language, etc.) being affected simultaneously [10, 12]. Research suggests that MCI generally develops into an Alzheimer's disease (AD) type of dementia. However, contradictory studies also support that MCI is reversible or could develop into non-AD type dementia [10, 29]. Therefore, to bring uniformity to the diagnosis of MCI, the international working group on MCI has given modified criteria for diagnosis, suggesting any cognitive impairment that fails to meet the diagnostic criteria of dementia is categorized as MCI [10].

2. MCI assessment

According to Petersen et al. [30], the clinician can use the progression criteria as per the description provided in the flowchart for an easy understanding of the procedure used for making a diagnosis for MCI. The same is depicted in **Figure 2** [31]. The clinician is thus faced with the challenge of evaluating this symptom, given that the patient appears with a cognitive concern. It is vital to obtain a patient's history and confirm it with someone who is familiar with the patient. It is critical that the patient, the patient's informant, or the physician expresses some level of cognitive concern. The cognitive concern is important since it reflects a change in the person's performance. MCI is not meant to reflect a person's low cognitive function for the rest of their life; rather, it is meant to show a shift in this specific person's cognitive function. As a result, the clinical history is vital in the absence of formal longitudinal

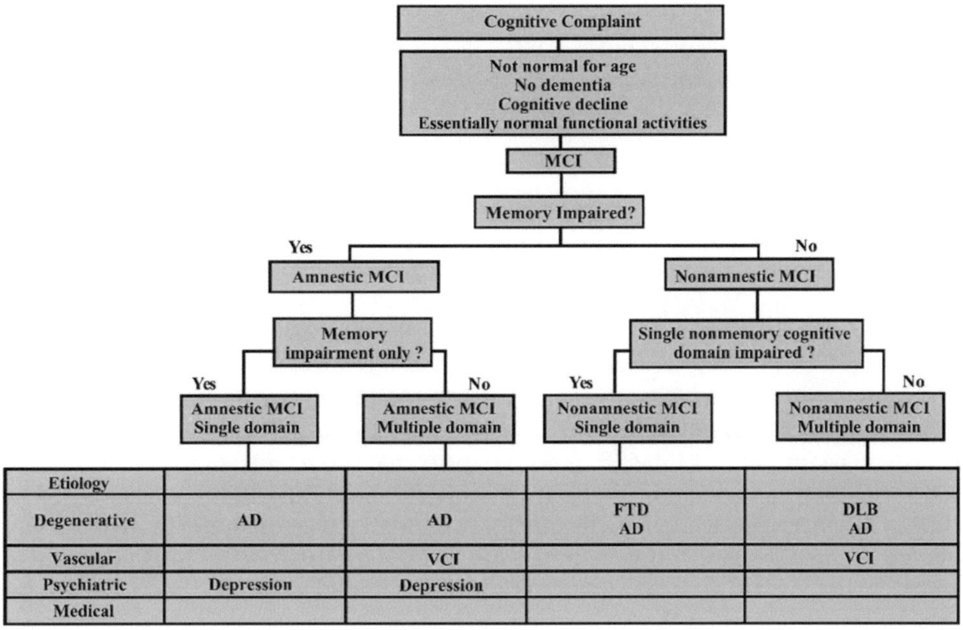

Figure 2.
Flowchart for clinical evaluation and diagnosis of cases with MCI.

cognitive data on an individual. The clinician should emphasize the types of cognitive changes the patient has experienced. If the primary concern is memory loss, the clinician should focus on recent forgetfulness occurrences (approximately in the last 6 months to a year). In cases of forgetfulness involving current events, appointments, visits by friends, or conversations, the physician should be particularly interested. If the patient begins to repeat themself, this indicates that impairments are emerging. Again, the clinician should evaluate for changes in that person's memory or cognitive performance [32].

The clinician should investigate the extent of the cognitive impairment. The question is whether the issue is solely about memory or does it also involve other cognitive areas like attention and concentration. Patients frequently identify cognitive alterations in the memory domain when, in reality, they may be referring to attention or language issues. It is essential to define the breadth of the cognitive shift. The clinician will need to conduct a mental status examination and explore the various cognitive domains at this time. If schedule allows, a mental status assessment using an instrument like the Montreal Cognitive Assessment (MoCA) or the Short Test of Mental Status can be useful, but the clinician should be aware that these screening instruments are insufficient to make the diagnosis; however, they can be useful in isolating domains of impairment and advising the clinician on additional assessments like neuroimaging and for amyloid imaging (MRI, PET scan, etc.,) and a CSF study [33, 34]. Neuropsychological testing can be beneficial if the key question with the patient is how to differentiate between the patient's symptoms and the changes in cognitive function that occur with normal aging. The neuropsychologist can examine whether the level of cognitive function is acceptable for the patient's age, gender, and education by describing the profile of cognitive function. If the clinician does not have access to this information, they must make the best assessment of function possible.

Test materials such as the Montreal Cognitive Assessment (MoCA) [34] and the Mini-Mental State Examination (MMSE) [35] are typically used to assess patients with cognitive impairment. According to Nasreddine et al. [34], the sensitivity of MMSE to detect MCI was only 18%, whereas the sensitivity of MoCA to detect MCI was 90% [34, 36]. The specificity of both tests was reported to be good. The poor sensitivity for the MMSE to see conditions of MCI was attributed to the poor scoring, and any score greater than 26 was considered normal, within which the scores of persons with MCI are just above average [37]. Hence, it can be concluded that the condition of MCI can be detected successfully using the MoCA.

Both MMSE and MoCA are primarily used for screening, and the time of administration required is 5–10 min. Subtle differences exist between the two. Longer delayed recall time and fewer trial learning stimuli are present in MoCA, giving more challenges to the patient. Executive and complex language abilities (abstraction) are not assessed in MMSE but in MoCA. This increases the complexity of the tasks of MoCA when compared to MMSE. Studies report that the attention tasks in MoCA, such as the digit span, sustained attention, and the serial 7 calculation task helped to discriminate between AD versus the normal and MCI group as all the three tasks were affected in the AD group but were preserved in MCI group. AD and MCI groups also demonstrated impairment in sentence repetition, and delayed recall was found to be the most impaired task in the MCI group [34].

With reference to the functional performance, a patient with MCI should suggest that the patient's daily function is mostly retained. However, the history of being assessed for any cognitive decline. For example, the patient may be inefficient at particular tasks and take longer to do them, but he or she will eventually be able to complete them without assistance. This form of evaluation satisfies the criteria retained for cognitive function requirements. This can be a very subjective judgment. Therefore, having a trustworthy informant on hand can help. However, if the individual continues to operate daily, such as driving, paying bills, and filing taxes, and appears normal to the casual observer, a function is often kept. Finally, the patient does not meet the criteria for dementia based on all of these factors. The person's cognitive deficits are not severe enough to interfere with daily activities. As a result, an essential condition for dementia is not met.

The clinician should then decide whether the patient has had a change in cognition, whether there is objective evidence of this, whether a function is generally intact, and whether or not the patient meets dementia criteria. Suppose MCI is considered to be a valid diagnosis. In that case, the clinician must then assess whether memory is a significant element of the cognitive impairment and if so, the amnestic MCI arms would be appropriate. The non-amnestic arm of the diagnosis, on the other hand, would apply if the person is experiencing cognitive loss, but their memory is generally intact.

Following the determination mentioned above of the clinical syndrome, the clinician must then discover the cause or etiology of the syndrome. **Figure 2** depicts potential explanations for various clinical symptoms with degenerative, vascular, psychiatric, or medical etiologies and can aid in determining the next steps in the diagnostic process. A degenerative disease is a plausible possibility if the onset of the disorder has been slow and gradual. A vascular contribution must also be evaluated if the patient has a history of vascular risk factors and has had cerebral ischemia episodes. Furthermore, some mental diseases, such as major depression or generalized anxiety disorder, might have cognitive components. As a result, cognition may be compromised in the early stages of these disorders. Other medical conditions, such as uncompensated heart failure, poorly controlled diabetes mellitus, or chronic obstructive pulmonary disease, must always be considered factors of cognitive impairment by the clinician. Some of these medical comorbidities are curable, and their drugs may also lead to clinical syndrome [32].

2.1 MCI pathogenesis and outcomes

An amyloid-b deposition is linked to dementia caused by decades of proteinopathy, such as Alzheimer's disease caused due to extraneuronal neuritic plaques and intracellularly neurofibrillary tangles. They are characterized as tauopathy for progressive supranuclear palsy, corticobasal degeneration, frontotemporal lobar degeneration, and synucleinopathy for Lewy body dementia and Parkinson's disease dementia. However, there are also significant aspects in the pathophysiology of dementia that can be modified, including a sedentary lifestyle, low nutritional status, social or environmental influences, and hereditary factors [38].

MCI can be caused by a variety of factors, including systemic disorders. Differential outcomes are caused by neurological diseases, drugs, and psychological disorders [39]. There are just a handful of possible outcomes of MCI—stabilization, progression, or reversion to normal aging. There is a unique presentation of metabolic disorders in older persons. Basic investigations are recommended, and when clinically necessary, neuroimaging is used. Reversible reasons are uncommon, with most cases occurring in surgical and depressive patients [32, 40–42].

If the clinician considers a degenerative condition the most likely cause, then the clinical symptoms can help identify an underlying diagnosis. If the patient has a typical amnestic condition with MCI and is in the right age range, Alzheimer's disease (AD) is a possible diagnosis. However, suppose the patient is having trouble with attention, concentration, and visuospatial difficulties. In that case, a form of dementia with Lewy body should be considered. If the person has behavioral changes, inappropriate behavior, apathy, lack of insight, and impaired attention and concentration, frontotemporal lobar degeneration should be considered. In fact, Alzheimer's disease, the most frequent degenerative disease of old age, can manifest itself in unusual ways involving attention, focus, and language [12, 32].

The clinician may be able to make a fair assumption about the nature of the condition based on the history and examination. Additional testing, such as an MRI scan, fluorodeoxyglucose positron emission tomography (FDG-PET) or positron emission tomography (PET) for amyloid imaging, and a CSF study, may be considered at this time. These additional tests may aid in determining the underlying cause of the clinical symptoms. While the US Food and Drug Administration (FDA) has not yet approved any pharmaceutical therapy for MCI caused by Alzheimer's disease, lifestyle changes and cognitive and behavioral therapies may be beneficial. Counseling patients about their expectations is also crucial. Medical comorbidities, such as sleep disorders like sleep apnea, should be investigated, as previously stated because some have curative components [12, 30, 32, 43].

3. MCI treatments

The FDA, the European Medicines Agency, and the Pharmaceuticals and Medical Devices Agency in Japan have not approved any pharmacological treatments for MCI. There have been numerous randomized control trials in the MCI spectrum, but none has been successful in slowing the progression of MCI to AD dementia [44–47]. The Alzheimer's Disease Cooperative Study tested donepezil with high-dose vitamin E in amnestic MCI as one of the earliest trials [32]. This study found that donepezil could delay the rate of advancement in all patients with amnestic MCI for the first year of the trial and perhaps for up to 2 years in those with amnestic MCI. They were positive for the APOE4 isoform. However, because the study was only supposed to last 36 months, no treatments were shown to be helpful at that point, and the trial was deemed a failure. Other studies employing cholinesterase inhibitors, which have been used to treat Alzheimer's disease dementia, have also failed [32, 44, 45].

Only a few research looked at the effects of over-the-counter (OTC) intervention on clinical MCI caused to Alzheimer's disease, according to a systematic review [37]. There are no studies that compare placebo to omega-3 fatty acids, soy, folic acid, B vitamin (folic acid plus B12), B vitamin (folic acid plus B6, B12), vitamin D plus calcium, vitamin E, vitamin C, or b-carotene in terms of MCI prevention. There was insufficient evidence to conclude the benefits of Ginkgo biloba, and a clinical trial found that multivitamins had no effect. In general, there is little evidence that OTC vitamins protect the brain [48].

There is research with reference to changes in lifestyle and non-pharmacologic therapy like aerobic exercise may be useful in slowing the progression of MCI to Dementia [49]. However, a 2010 state-of-the-science report from the National Institutes of Health (NIH) found no effective therapies for dementia progression [32]. However, recent evidence suggests that lifestyle adjustments may have some efficacy, which needs further investigation.

There was insufficient data to conclude the effect of a multi-component physical intervention that included flexibility, strength, balance, endurance, and aerobic training. No studies compared attention control to aerobic training, strength training, physical activity plus diet, physical activity plus protein supplement, or physical activity, diet, and cognitive training [37]. Even though single-component physical activity programs had negative results, a multidomain intervention appeared to improve cognitive function in older people with normal cognition. It is advised that clinicians encourage their patients to participate in clinical practice because the advantages can help avoid or manage other chronic conditions [50].

With reference to cognitive training, according to a systematic review, there is no clinical research on the protective impact of cognitive training in persons with normal cognitive function from developing MCI [37, 48]. Training in specific domains, such as reasoning, executive function/attention/processing speed, and memory, improved cognitive performance in the trained domains. As a result, there is inadequate evidence of cognitive training in people with the normal cognitive ability to prevent or delay cognitive decline [48].

4. Conclusion

In clinical practice and research, MCI has become an important topic. MCI established boundaries for this intermediate stage, focusing on earlier detection of incipient forms of cognitive impairments. Several randomized controlled studies for the MCI subtype caused by Alzheimer's disease are currently underway, and doctors should be aware of these research prospects for their patients. The cognitive abnormalities may be reversible once treatable etiologies of MCI (such as those caused by psychiatric illnesses, drugs, or medical comorbidities) are recognized. The development of biomarkers should give clinicians new tools for detecting and possibly treating MCI.

Conflict of interest

The authors report no conflicts of interest. The authors alone are responsible for the content and writing of the book chapter.

Funding

There is no funding by any agency for the manuscript.

Author details

Biraj Bhattarai[1*] and Hema Nagaraj[2]

1 Speech Language Pathologist Grade I, All India Institute of Speech and Hearing, Mysore, Karnataka, India

2 Assistant Professor, Department of Speech-Language Sciences, All India Institute of Speech and Hearing, Mysore, Karnataka, India

*Address all correspondence to: birajbhattarai29@gmail.com

IntechOpen

© 2022 The Author(s). Licensee IntechOpen. This chapter is distributed under the terms of the Creative Commons Attribution License (http://creativecommons.org/licenses/by/3.0), which permits unrestricted use, distribution, and reproduction in any medium, provided the original work is properly cited.

References

[1] DeCarli C, Massaro J, Harvey D, et al. Measures of brain morphology and infarction in the Framingham heart study: Establishing what is normal. Neurobiology of Aging. 2005;**26**:491-510. DOI: 10.1016/j.neurobiolaging.2004.05.004

[2] Raz N, Lindenberger U, Rodrigue KM, et al. Regional brain changes in aging healthy adults: General trends, individual differences and modifiers. Cerebral Cortex. 2005;**15**:1676-1689. DOI: 10.1093/cercor/bhi044

[3] Ylikoski A, Erkinjuntti T, Raininko R, et al. White matter hyperintensities on MRI in the neurologically nondiseased elderly: Analysis of cohorts of consecutive subjects aged 55 to 85 years living at home. Stroke. 1995;**26**:1171-1177. DOI: 10.1161/01.STR.26.7.1171

[4] Kral VA. Senescent forgetfulness: Benign and malignant. Canadian Medical Association Journal. 1962;**86**:257-260

[5] Crook T, Bartus RT, Ferris SH, et al. Age-associated memory impairment: Proposed diagnostic criteria and measures of clinical change—Report of a National Institute of Mental Health work group. Developmental Neuropsychology. 1986;**2**:261-276. DOI: 10.1080/87565648609540348

[6] Ritchie K, Touchon J. Mild cognitive impairment: Conceptual basis and current nosological status. Lancet. 2000;**355**:225-228

[7] Bell CC. DSM-IV: Diagnostic and statistical manual of mental disorders. Journal of American Medical Association. 1994;**272**:828. DOI: 10.1001/jama.1994.03520100096046

[8] Williams KN, Kemper S. Interventions to reduce cognitive decline in aging. Journal of psychosocial nursing and mental health services. 2010;**48**(5):42-51. DOI: 10.3928/02793695-20100331-03

[9] Fillit HM, Butler RN, O'Connell AW, Albert MS, Birren JE, Cotman CW, et al. Achieving and maintaining cognitive vitality with aging. Mayo Clinic Proceedings. 2002;**77**(7):681-696. DOI: 10.4065/77.7.681

[10] Anand R, Chapman SB, Zientz J, Toussaint K. Mild cognitive impairment: A clinical perspective. Perspect Gerontology. 2005;**10**:10-14. DOI: 10.1044/gero10.2.10

[11] Grundman M, Petersen RC, Ferris SH, et al. Mild cognitive impairment can be distinguished from Alzheimer disease and Normal aging for clinical trials. Archives of Neurology. 2004;**61**:59-66. DOI: 10.1001/archneur.61.1.59

[12] Petersen RC. Mild cognitive impairment as a diagnostic entity. Journal of Internal Medicine. 2004;**256**(3):183-194. DOI: 10.1111/j.1365-2796.2004.01388.x

[13] O'Brien JT, Erkinjuntti T, Reisberg B, et al. Vascular cognitive impairment. Lancet Neurology. 2003;**2**:89-98

[14] McKhann GM, Knopman DS, Chertkow H, Hyman BT, Jack CR, Jr, Kawas CH, et al. The diagnosis of dementia due to Alzheimer's disease: Recommendations from the National Institute on Aging-Alzheimer's association workgroups on diagnostic guidelines for Alzheimer's disease. Alzheimer's & Dementia: The journal of the Alzheimer's Association. 2011;**7**(3):263-269. DOI: 10.1016/j.jalz.2011.03.005

[15] Wilson RS, Aggarwal NT, Barnes LL, et al. Cognitive decline in incident

Alzheimer disease in a community population. Neurology. 2010;**74**:951-955. DOI: 10.1212/WNL.0b013e3181d64786

[16] Price JL. Diagnostic criteria for Alzheimer's disease. Neurobiology of Aging. 1997;**18**(4 Suppl):S67–S70. DOI: 10.1016/S0197-4580(97)00072-9

[17] Bennett DA, Schneider JA, Arvanitakis Z, et al. Neuropathology of older persons without cognitive impairment from two community-based studies. Neurology. 2006;**66**:1837-1844. DOI: 10.1212/01.WNL.0000219668.47116.E6

[18] Amieva H, Jacqmin-Gadda H, Orgogozo JM, et al. The 9 year cognitive decline before dementia of the Alzheimer type: A prospective population-based study. Brain. 2005;**128**:1093-1101. DOI: 10.1093/BRAIN/AWH451

[19] Flicker C, Ferris SH, Reisberg B. Mild cognitive impairment in the elderly: Predictors of dementia. Neurology. 1991;**41**(7):1006-1006

[20] Petersen RC. Mild Cognitive Impairment: Aging to Alzheimer's Disease. United States: Oxford University Press; 2003

[21] Petersen RC, Stevens JC, Ganguli M, et al. Practice parameter: Early detection of dementia: Mild cognitive impairment (an evidence-based review). Neurology. 2001;**56**:1133-1142. DOI: 10.1212/WNL.56.9.1133

[22] Rountree SD, Waring SC, Chan WC, et al. Importance of subtle amnestic and nonamnestic deficits in mild cognitive impairment: Prognosis and conversion to dementia. Dementia and Geriatric Cognitive Disorders. 2007;**24**:476-482. DOI: 10.1159/000110800

[23] Murman DL. The impact of age on cognition. Seminars in Hearing. 2015;**36**(3):111-121. DOI: 10.1055/s-0035-1555115

[24] Cloutier S, Chertkow H, Kergoat MJ, Gauthier S, Belleville S. Patterns of cognitive decline prior to dementia in persons with mild cognitive impairment. Journal of Alzheimer's Disease. 2015;**47**(4):901-913. DOI: 10.3233/JAD-142910. PMID: 26401770; PMCID: PMC4923749

[25] Ebly EM, Parhad IM, Hogan DB, Fung TS. Prevalence and types of dementia in the very old: Results from the Canadian Study of Health and Aging. Neurology 1994;**44**:1593-600. DOI: 10.1001/archneur.1995.00540300086018

[26] Lopez OL. Mild cognitive impairment. Continuum (Minneap Minn). 2013 Apr;**19**(2 Dementia):411-24. DOI: 10.1212/01.CON.0000429175.29601.97. PMID: 23558486, PMCID: PMC3915547

[27] Tierney MC, Szalai JP, Snow WG, Fisher RH, Nores A, Nadon G, et al. Prediction of probable Alzheimer's disease in memory-impaired patients: A prospective longitudinal study. Neurology. 1996;**46**(3):661-665. DOI: 10.1212/WNL.46.3.661

[28] Jorm AF, Christensen H, Korten AE, et al. Do cognitive complaints either predict future cognitive decline or reflect past cognitive decline? A longitudinal study of an elderly community sample. Psychological Medicine. 1997;**27**:91-98. DOI: 10.1017/S0033291796003923

[29] Gauthier S, Touchon J. Mild cognitive impairment is not a clinical entity and should not be treated. Archives of Neurology. 2005. DOI: 10.1001/archneur.62.7.1164

[30] Petersen RC, Caracciolo B, Brayne C, et al. Mild cognitive impairment: A

concept in evolution. Journal of Internal Medicine. 2014;**275**:214-228. DOI: 10.1111/joim.12190

[31] Kramer JH, Nelson A, Johnson JK, et al. Multiple cognitive deficits in amnestic mild cognitive impairment. Dementia and Geriatric Cognitive Disorders. 2006. DOI: 10.1159/000095303

[32] Petersen RC. Mild cognitive impairment. Neurology. 2016;**22**:404-418

[33] Weiner MW, Veitch DP, Aisen PS, et al. Impact of the Alzheimer's Disease Neuroimaging Initiative, 2004 to 2014. Alzheimers Dement. 2015;**11**:865-884. DOI: 10.1016/J.JALZ.2015.04.005

[34] Nasreddine ZS, Phillips NA, Bédirian V, et al. The Montreal cognitive assessment, MoCA: A brief screening tool for mild cognitive impairment. Journal of the American Geriatrics Society. 2005;**53**:695-699. DOI: 10.1111/j.1532-5415.2005.53221.x

[35] Folstein MF, Folstein SE, McHugh PR. "Mini-mental state". A practical method for grading the cognitive state of patients for the clinician. Journal of Psychiatric Research. 1975. DOI: 10.1016/0022-3956(75)90026-6

[36] Tsai JC, Chen CW, Chu H, et al. Comparing the sensitivity, specificity, and predictive values of the Montreal cognitive assessment and Mini-mental state examination when screening people for mild cognitive impairment and dementia in Chinese population. Archives of Psychiatric Nursing. 2016;**30**:486-491. DOI: 10.1016/J.APNU.2016.01.015

[37] Jongsiriyanyong S, Limpawattana P. Mild cognitive impairment in clinical practice: A review article. American Journal of Alzheimer's Disease and Other Dementias. 2018;**33**:500-507. DOI: 10.1177/1533317518791401

[38] Honig LS. Translational research in neurology: Dementia. Archives of Neurology. 2012;**69**:969-977

[39] Jack CR, Petersen RC, Xu YC, et al. Prediction of AD with MRI-based hippocampal volume in mild cognitive impairment. Neurology. 1999. DOI: 10.1212/wnl.52.7.1397

[40] Ganguli M, Fu B, Snitz BE, et al. Mild cognitive impairment: Incidence and vascular risk factors in a population-based cohort. Neurology. 2013;**80**:2112-2120. DOI: 10.1212/WNL.0B013E318295D776

[41] Sachdev PS, et al. Factors predicting reversion from mild cognitive impairment to normal cognitive functioning: A population-based study. PLoS One. 2013;**8**(3):e59649. DOI: 10.1371/journal.pone.0059649

[42] Koepsell TD, Monsell SE. Reversion from mild cognitive impairment to normal or near-normal cognition: Risk factors and prognosis. Neurology. 2012;**79**:1591-1598. DOI: 10.1212/WNL.0B013E31826E26B7

[43] Petersen RC, Smith GE, Waring SC, et al. Mild cognitive impairment: Clinical characterization and outcome. Archives of Neurology. 1999;**56**:303-308. DOI: 10.1001/archneur.56.3.303

[44] Doody RS, Ferris SH, Salloway S, et al. Donepezil treatment of patients with MCI: A 48-week randomized, placebo-controlled trial. Neurology. 2009;**72**:1555-1561. DOI: 10.1212/01.WNL.0000344650.95823.03

[45] Feldman HH, Ferris S, Winblad B, et al. Effect of rivastigmine on delay to diagnosis of Alzheimer's disease from mild cognitive impairment: The InDDEx study. Lancet Neurology. 2007;**6**:501-512. DOI: 10.1016/S1474-4422(07)70109-6

[46] Petersen RC, Thomas RG, Grundman M, et al. Vitamin E and donepezil for the treatment of mild cognitive impairment. The New England Journal of Medicine. 2005;**352**:361. DOI: 10.1056/NEJMOA050151

[47] Thal LJ, Ferris SH, Kirby L, et al. A randomized, double-blind, study of rofecoxib in patients with mild cognitive impairment. Neuropsychopharmacology. 2005;**30**:1204-1215. DOI: 10.1038/SJ.NPP.1300690

[48] Butler M, Nelson VA, Davila H, et al. Over-the-counter supplement interventions to prevent cognitive decline, mild cognitive impairment, and clinical Alzheimer-type dementia. Annals of Internal Medicine. 2018;**168**:52-62

[49] Lautenschlager NT, Cox KL, Flicker L, et al. Effect of physical activity on cognitive function in older adults at risk for Alzheimer disease: A randomized trial. Journal of American Medical Association. 2008;**300**:1027-1037. DOI: 10.1001/jama.300.9.1027

[50] Brasure M, Desai P, Davila H, et al. Physical activity interventions in preventing cognitive decline and Alzheimer-type dementia: A systematic review. Annals of Internal Medicine. 2018;**168**:30-38. DOI: 10.7326/M17-1528

Chapter 9

Methods of Treating Autism: Holistic Approach to the Rehabilitation of People with the Spectrum of Autism

Elzbieta Trylinska-Tekielska, Dorota Pietraszewska, Iwona Stanisawska and Ada Holak

Abstract

In recent years, the autism spectrum in children has been increasingly recognized. Parental awareness and the knowledge of health professionals are critical to the early diagnosis of autistic disorders. The autism spectrum disorder (ASD) is a complex neurodevelopmental disorder. The diagnosis of autism spectrum disorders is made on the basis of observation of behavior in three areas: social interaction, communication, and behavioral rigidity. The most common diagnosis is in children around 2–5 years of age, but the autism spectrum can be diagnosed at any age, also in adulthood. As the spectrum of autism varies, symptoms of autism may differ slightly from person to person. In order to exclude the presence of ASD in a child or adult, it is necessary to diagnose with the use of various tools, in which both a psychologist-diagnostician and a psychiatrist are involved. After diagnosis, the next important step is to include therapeutic and rehabilitation activities aimed at improving the functioning of the individual in disturbed areas. Lack of proper rehabilitation may lead to profound functional disturbances at a later age.

Keywords: spectrum autism, diagnosis, symptoms, methods of rehabilitation, therapy

1. Introduction

The word autism comes from the Greek autós, which means "alone." The concept was introduced into psychiatry in 1911 by the Swiss psychiatrist Eugen Bleuler for the inability to maintain relations with the environment. The first description of a person with autism was made in 1943 by psychiatrist Leo Kanner. Autism spectrum disorders (ASDs) are characterized by disturbances in the ability to communicate feelings and build interpersonal relationships, impoverishment and stereotypical behavior, and difficulties in integrating sensory impressions. According to the ICD 11 classification in force in Poland since 2022, there is a wider diagnosis of autism spectrum disorders, which combines the categories of childhood autism, atypical autism, and Asperger syndrome described earlier in ICD-10 into one main category of Autism Spectrum Disorder (ASD) included in the chapter on neurodevelopmental disorders. ASD is described in seven different variants listed as follows:

6A02 Autism Spectrum Disorder
6A02.0 Autism spectrum disorder without intellectual development disorder and with mild or no functional language impairment
6A02.1 Autism spectrum disorder with mental development disorder and mild or no functional language impairment
6A02.2 Autism spectrum disorder without impaired intellectual development and with impaired functional language
6A02.3 Autism spectrum disorder with impaired intellectual development and functional disorders
6A02.4 Autism spectrum disorder without intellectual development disorder and lack of functional language
6A02.5 Autism spectrum disorder with impaired intellectual development and lack of functional language
6A02.Y Other specified autism spectrum disorders
6A02.Z Autism spectrum disorder, unspecified [1]

Most people with ASD exhibit features that impair functioning in three areas: communication, social, and behavioral (the so-called autism spectrum triad). The triad of disorders distinguished by Wing and Gould [2] is reflected in the current DSM V classification, which lists the following symptoms important in the diagnosis of ASD:

1. shortcomings in human development, especially in the capacity to participate in alternating social interactions,

2. deficits and dysfunctions in communication (verbal and nonverbal),

3. the presence of rigid patterns of behavior, activity, and interests.

An important element added to the diagnostic criteria in DSM-5 is the inclusion of disturbances within the sensory profile.

Symptoms of autism are most often seen in early childhood, but may not be fully manifested until social expectations exceed the child's limited abilities. It should be emphasized that autism is not a mental illness. It has been assumed that the underlying causes are errors in neurological development, i.e., abnormalities in the formation of the central nervous system, starting in the prenatal age.

For proper therapy, it is also important to determine the severity of symptoms and their impact on the daily functioning of people with ASD:

L1 —patient and family require support —problems mainly relate to social relations,
L2 —requires significant support —communication problems with people,
L3 —requires very significant support —incapable of verbal and nonverbal communication [3].

2. Diagnosing ASD

Autism spectrum disorders are multifactorial disorders, and its exact causes are not fully understood. Due to the very different manifestation of symptoms, diagnosing autism spectrum disorders is a complex process, consisting of several stages and requiring the cooperation of a team of specialists. The word "spectrum" means that each person with autism is different, and each person with autism manifests itself in a different set of characteristics and their severity. Despite the neurobiological basis of autism spectrum disorders, there are still no biological indicators that would allow them to be used in everyday clinical diagnosis [4]. The diagnosis of ASD remains a clinical diagnosis, based on the observation and assessment of the patient's behavior and cognitive functions. The disorder long-term affects a person's ability to take care of himself, participate in society. The diagnosis of ASD also affects other family members of a person with ASD [5, 6].

Although there is no single conclusive test or biological marker for ASD detection, there are many screening and diagnostic tools that can be used in the examination of children with suspected neurodevelopmental disorders [4].

2.1 Diagnostic tools

2.1.1 CHAT

Screening tools available include "first-level" tests that can be used during your primary care physician visit, including the Checklist for Autism in Toddlers (CHAT; parental assessment/physician observation; examination of children between 18 and 24 months of age) [4]. This tool is intended for testing 18-month-old children during pediatric follow-up visits, although it can also be used for older children—up to 24 and even 36 months of age. This tool consists of two parts: nine questions asked to parents and five short clinical trials. CHAT has a consistent and fairly well-documented theoretical basis. CHAT is recommended to pediatricians in Great Britain by National Autistic Society. One of the versions of CHAT is M-CHAT (Modified-CHAT) intended for testing children aged 16–30 months [7]. This questionnaire contains 23 questions (nine were taken directly from CHAT) and is completed by the parents. Another variation of CHAT is Q-CHAT (Quantitative CHecklist for Autism in Toddlers) intended for the study of children aged 18–24 months. In the questionnaire, the parent assesses the frequency of a given behavior or the severity of the problem on a five-point scale (not a dichotomous one, unlike M-CHAT) [8].

In Western countries and the United States, autism is the most frequently used interviewing tool Diagnostic Interview–Revised (ADI-R). The Polish version has been available recently thanks to Dr. Izabela Chojnicka, who is the author of the Polish language version [9].

2.1.2 ADI-R

It is a diagnostic tool used to conduct an interview. Its publisher is Western Psychological Services. Initially, it was used for research purposes. It is now a "*Comprehensive, standardized, and partially structured interview that is conducted with parents or guardians people with ASD*" [9].

During its development, the currently applicable diagnostic criteria ICD-10 and DSM-IV-TR were taken into account. It is recommended for children from 24 months of mental age. It consists of 93 items grouped into the following headings:

Introduction and introductory questions – a section consisting of six items concerning the family situation, the process of education and treatment, diagnosis.
Early development – a section of seven items concerning the onset of symptoms of milestones in development and purity training.
Acquisition and loss of skills, including language skills – section consisting of 20 items.
Language and functioning of communication – a department consisting of 21 items.
Social development and fun – a department consisting of 17 items.
Behaviors and interests – section consisting of 13 items.
General behavior – a section of 14 items.
Final comments – a section consisting of three items concerning incl. Impressions of the interviewer [9].

The interview lasts from 1.5 to 4 hours depending on the age of the child. The individual items refer to both the previous behavior and the current behavior. The interview also includes questions about the presence of some symptoms typical of other pervasive development disorders, some questions about behaviors that are less important in the diagnosis of the autism spectrum but show the specificity of development of many children. The questionnaire also includes questions about the family or previous diagnoses and the course of any previous therapy. The scoring is nine levels, each question is assessed, and the diagnosis is made on the basis of an algorithm.

ADI-R interview may differ from the clinical diagnosis, but it is a very helpful tool in making a diagnosis, and it helps to gather a large amount of information.

> *"When reading Western scientific publications, especially in the field of autism spectrum biology, there are no studies in which the diagnosis of the respondents would not be made on the basis of ADI-R and ADOS-G" [9].*

2.2 Behavior observation scales

2.2.1 ADOS

It is a tool for direct observation of behavior. It is standardized and consists of four protocols differing in terms of age and stage of speech development. It is most often used with the ADI-R. This tool consists of a number of experimental situations in which the observer is also a participant.

2.2.2 CARS

This scale is useful for the observation of children from 0 to 16 years of age; however, it should be noted that its effectiveness is greater for children from 2 years of age. It includes 15 areas of behavioral behavior, information comes from parents or other people staying with the child. The CARS scale is commonly used for treatment planning and assessment of progress [10].

DOI: http://dx.doi.org/10.5772/intechopen.105435

2.2.3 PEP-R

PEP-R is a useful and popular tool for the functional diagnosis of a child. It is used in designing the therapy of a child with developmental problems. Thanks to the PEP-R test, it is possible to assess the educational needs of the child and determine the baseline level for therapy.

The PEP-R test consists of two parts: the developmental scale and the behavioral scale.

The scale of development allows for the assessment of the child's functioning in the following areas:

Limitation, perception, fine and gross motor skills, eye-hand coordination, cognitive activities, and communication. It consists of 131 tasks in total.

The behavior scale is designed to identify responses and behaviors. The degree of disorders and the areas in which these disorders appear are assessed. The behavior scale consists of 42 tasks divided into four areas: networking and emotional reactions, play and interest in objects, reactions to stimuli, and speech [10–12].

3. The multifactorial basis of autism spectrum disorders

The autism spectrum is much more than diagnostic criteria. So the difference between defining autism spectrum disorder (ASD) and developmental pattern (ASC) is analogous to the difference between negative and positive definitions of health. In the first case, we focus on deficits and looking for therapeutic measures to help mask them. In the second case, we focus on the resources of the individual, resulting from its proper development pattern, and we look for ways to strengthen it. According to Baron-Cohen, there are currently four narratives describing the autism spectrum: disorder, disability, difference, and disease. However, it was the terms "otherness" and "disability" that he indicated as fully compatible with the concept of neurodiversity understood as nature's strategy aimed at ensuring the scope of the human species (human minds) with a variety of challenges inherent in different environments (Baron-Cohen 2020: 138). Thus, this position can be considered more akin to the treatment of the autism spectrum as a developmental pattern than as a disorder. It is worth quoting at this point the opinion of one of the Polish researchers: "The spectrum of autism is a borderline category in many respects, blurred and unclear, ephemeral and changeable, and thus constantly revealing its arbitrariness and more social than biological construction" [5].

The state of knowledge about autism does not give unequivocal answers as to the causes of this disorder. The development of neurobiology and neuroimaging prompted many researchers to seek answers to the question of where does autism come from in neurological areas. Intensive efforts are underway to elucidate the neurobiology of autism. The combination of neuroanatomical abnormalities revealed in children's brain MRI studies with abnormalities in neuropsychic development and autistic symptoms seems to be of particular interest. Significant links were found between autism spectrum disorders and the presence of certain biomarkers. For example, functional resonance in children with autism shows that human facial image processing takes place in a different area than in healthy people; autistic people look at human faces, paying attention to the mouth area, not the eye area. In his works, Tuchmann [13] showed that various types of EEG abnormalities often occur in the group of ASD patients. About 20% of ASD patients in basal resting EEG display show epileptic activity mainly in the form of focal lesions (spikes). EEG tests performed during sleep show even more seizure disorders in children with ASD. The EEG test is a method that can be used to assess the work of the brain in children with autism. However, there are no typical EEG patterns that would be unambiguous and specific to an ASD image.

Another hypothesis that contributes to the search for the causes of ASD is the theory of mirror neurons. The broken mirror hypothesis assumes that there is abnormal mirror cell activity in the brain of autistic people. Mirror cells are responsible for the mental mapping of motor activities, emotions, and sensory experiences observed in other people. In people with autism spectrum disorders, decreased activity of these cells in the area of the inferior frontal gyrus may explain the inability to understand the intentions of other people, in the insula and anterior part of the cingulate gyrus—difficulties in understanding emotional states, and in the angular gyrus—language disorders [14]. Oberman et al. [15], by monitoring mi waves in the EEG record, proved that in people with the autism spectrum, the activity of mirror neurons in the premotor cortex is reduced. These waves are attenuated by the discharges of motor neurons when making conscious body movements and by discharging mirror neurons when observing these movements in others. In children on the autism spectrum, mu-wave suppression is not observed when observing the movements of other people, which confirms the low activity of mirror neurons [16].

It seems interesting to analyze the relationship between symptoms of autism and possible dysfunctions in various regions of the brain. It is known that the centers located in different lobes of the cerebral cortex are responsible for higher mental functions. The temporal lobe is responsible for speech, remembering, verbal memory, object recognition, musical hearing and sound sensation, and smell analysis. Damage to the temporal lobes results in impaired hearing, speech understanding and sound perception, impaired selective attention to auditory and visual stimuli, problems with recognizing and describing the seen objects, and difficulties in recognizing the face (prosopagnosia). Functional disorders in the left hemisphere impede the ordering and categorization of verbal information and are responsible for difficulties in understanding speech (Wernicke's aphasia). On the other hand damage to the right hemisphere can cause speech orthosis. Centers in the temporal lobe are responsible for problems related to recall, disorders of sexual behavior, and control of aggressive behavior. Speech abnormalities of various degrees are evident in people suffering from autism spectrum disorders. They are of various dimensions and quality, ranging from a complete lack of speech understanding, through speech that is exclusively echolalia and does not serve the communicative function, through semi-communicative speech, poor to almost normal active speech, characterized by impaired prosody, intonation and a weak pragmatic meaning of language. What is typical in the picture of autistic disorders is also frequent aggressive and auto-aggressive behaviors, which are an expression of the dysfunction of the right temporal lobe. Therefore, in people suffering from autism, dysfunctions of the frontal and prefrontal areas are typical, which is manifested in the presented symptoms: stereotypical behavior and interests, disturbed social interactions, lack of understanding and socioemotional reciprocity. An important function is also played by the limbic lobe, which is responsible not only for the analysis of olfactory sensations and pain, but also for controlling negative emotions, focusing attention, memory, and learning. The manifestation of dysfunction in this area of the brain in people on the autism spectrum is hyperactivity, psychomotor restlessness, severe attention and memory disorders, loss of control over emotions, as well as disorders in the area of sensory integration (hypersensitivity or hypersensitivity to pain, touch, sounds) [17].

F. Warren, director of the National Association for Children and Adults with Autism in the United States, describes the symptoms of autism spectrum disorder in this way, making the far-reaching thesis that autism is caused by damage to the brain. "The symptoms of autism are caused by damage to the brain and include: disturbances and delays in mastering the habits of daily living, social and language habits .... These children have an abnormal reaction. This applies to both individual senses and the entire group. This applies to sight, hearing, touch, pain, sense of balance, taste, smell, and also to body posture ... Speech and linguistic development are delayed or completely absent in these children. There may also be specific thinking abilities. In speech, we observe an incorrect accent, a limited understanding of concepts, the use of words in such a way that they are not associated with things that mean (...) abnormal ways of contacting people, objects and situations (...) they do not react properly to adults as well as peers. They also do not use objects and toys in the usual way (...). Autism occurs as a single disorder or in combination with others that damage the functions of the brain: viral infections, metabolic disorders or epilepsy" [18].

4. The nutritional aspect of the autism spectrum

Etiopathogenesis of these disorders is multifactorial, and both predispositions are important genetic, factors environmental-like and factors related to answer layout immune system and functioning cable alimentary [19, 20]. With spectrum disorder autism, gastrointestinal symptoms often coexist. It is suspected that children with autism spectrum disorders may suffer from improper digestion of gluten proteins and casein, leading to the formation of peptides that may act as endogenous opioids (including milk caso–morphin- and gluten-based gliadomorphins), influencing the functioning of the central system nervous [21, 22]. Gastrointestinal symptoms in children with ASD may also be caused by hypochloridia and decreased secretion of gastric acid, less activity of amylolytic enzymes, intestinal disaccharidases, and inflammation of the esophagus, stomach or intestines. In this case, children with ASD suffer from autoimmune diseases and diseases, including celiac disease [23]. Increased permeability of the intestinal mucosa and imbalance of the intestinal microflora are also more frequent in patients with autism spectrum disorders occurrence increased permeability membranes mucous bowels and imbalance of the intestinal microflora [24, 25]. Research conducted in 2018, which drew attention to the importance of dietary ingredients and their impact on the somatic behavior of children with ASD, clearly documented positive changes in groups subjected to specific diets.

In children with ASD before the elimination diet, the parents more often observed gastrointestinal symptoms, especially flatulence, abdominal pain and diarrhea ($p \leq 0.05$) (**Table 1**), more often than in children who did not undergo dietary modification (**Table 1**). Most children experience these symptoms they gave way after introduction diets elimination [19, 26]. They write about the advantages and disadvantages of nutritional treatment of the autism spectrum disorder (based on their research) and emphasize that in some cases GFCF (gluten-free, casein-free) diets - ketogenic, low-phenol, low-oxalate may even cause the disappearance of disorders, symptoms characteristic of ASD. Parents of these children observe the beneficial effects: children sleep better, learn faster, blood results improve, rashes disappear. Perseverance behavior is also reduced. [27] Among ASD patients, deficiencies of vitamins B, C, K, and D3 and elements—calcium, potassium, and iron—are common. Deficiency of these ingredients may negatively affect the functioning of the neurological system.

Symptoms	Children with ASD			
	On elimination diet n = 27		On usual diet n = 23v	
	In the past	At present	In the past	At present
Reux	22		4	
Vomiting	37	7	22	
Atulence	59	30	13	
Bellyache	30		22	
Abdominal pain	59	22	13	9
Diarrhea	67	19	30	
Constipation	48	22	61	39

Source: Probl Hig Epidemiol 2018, 99 (1): 12–20.

Table 1.
Gastrointestinal tract symptoms in children with autism spectrum disorders in the past and at present (%).

Adequate supply of omega-3 fatty acids and probiotics may have a positive effect on the condition of patients with ASD [28].

5. Relation of the therapist —the parent of a child from the autism spectrum

The assumptions of working with ASD people say, first of all, about establishing a good relationship with this person. A very important element in building such a relationship is creating a safe space in which we will work with a person with ASD, developing a way of communication and supporting the family of a person with ASD.

One of the most important elements of the development of a child with autism—apart from family adaptation—is properly selected and continued specialist and home therapy. A specialist or a group of specialists should work with the child, who will first of all give the correct diagnosis and repeat it, tracking the child's development and adjusting the therapy to the changes in the child's behavior and its health. It is very important that parents have a full understanding of current and changing techniques regarding the care, care and development of an autism spectrum child in everyday life. At this stage, the exchange of experiences between parents and mutual support both in sharing their perceptions and experiences, as well as the need to obtain help is very important. [29].

Cooperation in the parent-therapist relationship allows parents to participate in the child's therapy and get to know them better, notice characteristic behaviors or progress that they do not notice in the home environment. The best results are achieved when the therapy starts in early childhood, when the child receives the most stimuli, develops the fastest, and the parents are strongly involved in cooperation to obtain the best results. Parents' participation in the child's therapy combines the specialist's experience with parental care, which brings the best results [30].

Pisula illustrates this on the example of the TEACCH model, in which it was assumed that parents learn how to cooperate with a child from therapists, and therapists get to know the child through the prism of the parent. It is a model of mutual support in everyday functioning. The better prepared the parents are, the better the results are achieved by working with the child at home, which has a positive effect

DOI: http://dx.doi.org/10.5772/intechopen.105435

not only on the child, but also on the whole family. Parents finally take control of the situation and stop being helpless about the behavior of their autistic child [30].

The best results are to stick to a few basic rules, starting with the fact that it should be remembered that the family has the greatest influence on the child's development and that it is the basis for his progress and should spend the most time on exercise, maintaining routine, rhythm, noting behavior changes. Certainly, a specialist or a group of specialists who exchange information and observations with parents on an ongoing basis should work with an autistic child. It is important to adjust the family's capabilities and resources, to pay attention to how to cope with their situation, and to establish solid relationships with other families operating under similar circumstances.

In addition to the great role of the parent, it should be remembered that it is the specialist's task to get to know the child and the conditions of his family, its strengths and weaknesses, and strive to cooperate with the child's parents, enabling its development to the fullest extent. Developing a relationship with the parents is as important a goal for the therapist as the work with the child itself. Thanks to this, the therapist inspires confidence in parents, which has a positive effect on the proposals of various solutions on his part. Otherwise, with a poor relationship with the parents, they may react negatively to his methods [31].

6. Therapeutic methods and techniques

Autism is a way of human development different from the typical one, manifested by differences in the way of communication, establishing relationships, expressing emotions, learning, and a diverse pattern of behavior. Each person with autism is an individual, and the abovementioned features may be of varying intensity. Autism accompanies a person throughout his life. After 6 years of analyzes, the NAC (National Autism Center) report was published, summarizing the research on the therapy of children, adolescents, and adults with autism. Its main goal is to select those forms of therapy that are most effective based on reliable scientific evidence. 2015 NAC report prepared as a result of the analysis of 361 scientific studies on methods of therapy for people with ASD. The report divided the treatments used into three groups: established (scientifically proven with strong and abundant evidence for their effectiveness), promising (there is evidence for the effectiveness of the method, but too little research is conducted), and undefined (very little or no evidence of a positive effect of the method). The established therapeutic methods are: behavioral methods, cognitive-behavioral interventions, modeling, natural teaching models, social skills training, activity plans. The group of promising therapies includes: alternative and supportive communication, relationship therapy, desensitization training, rehabilitation, massage, language training (resource and understanding), interventions based on new technology, therapies based on Theory of Mind Training, PECS, and music therapy. The group of undetermined therapies includes auditory training, the method of facilitated communication, gluten-free and casein-free diets, sensory integration, and additionally zootherapies or electroconvulsive therapies.

6.1 Physiotherapy

Each child diagnosed with an autism spectrum disorder or other related pervasive development disorder also has its own individual range of problems and dysfunctions. Their degree of intensity is also varied, which results in an absolute need for individualization of therapy. The therapeutic program must take into account the personality of the patient, as well as his current abilities and needs. It is important that the working methods used do not eliminate each other, but work complementary and synergistically, only then can they effectively activate the child's development. The current tendencies in the world's leading autism spectrum therapy centers dictate the broadly understood complexity of the actions of specialized institutions on children affected by the autism spectrum. This means that institutions that deal with the treatment of pervasive disorders should create and implement comprehensive rehabilitation programs, which should be arranged in the field of rehabilitation, therapy, vocational and general education, and social care. Not only every child needs therapeutic support, but also his family (siblings, parents, grandparents, and other people) who have close contact with the child.

The impacts of specialized institutions on patients with the autism spectrum can be divided into:

- medical/medical: differential diagnosis (medical interview, examination, direct observation), symptomatological, causal (specialist examinations, including: EEG, CT, immunological panel, metabolic panel, genetic tests, endoscopic examinations, loads, deficiencies), biomedical therapy (elimination diets, detoxification, chelation, supplementation, strengthening the immune system), pharmacotherapy,

- psychological: psychometric tests, direct observation, analysis of video materials, functional diagnosis, therapeutic programs for work at home, psychoeducation, general rehabilitation programs, training, workshops, support groups and family psychotherapy, Video Home Training,

- educational/pedagogical: educational leveling, general education programs, implementation of programs based on various working methods (behavioral method, Doman's method, Delacato method, activity albums method, TEACCH, options method and others),

- communication: proper speech therapy (speech evocation and articulation correction), facilitated communication (pictograms, PECES), nonverbal communication training,

- social: emergency care, 24-hour care (boarding house, hostel), living and financial support, legal support for the family,

- therapeutic: neurorehabilitation, manual techniques (cranial therapy, microkinesitherapy, classic surface, and deep massage), integration therapy (group music therapy, Sherborne developing movement, art therapy, creative therapy, occupational therapy, good start method), relational therapy (dog therapy, hippotherapy, therapy by contact with a horse or a dolphin or a cat), sensory revalidation/sensuum revalidatio (monosensory therapy, polysensory therapy, sensory integration, sequential therapy, individual music therapy, auditory training with the Tomatis method, therapy based on liquid and loose materials, Knill therapy, Masgut method, relaxation, hydrotherapy, work in the darkroom, therapy in the room for experiencing the world, Affolter assisted movement method [32].

In short, it can be said that medical interactions are primarily aimed at eliminating or minimizing the causes of disturbed CNS activity, as well as at improving the somatic state of the patient. Psychological support is needed to assess the level of a child's functioning in various areas, to set directions for further influence, and to monitor the progress made. The work of psychologists in autism spectrum therapy is also used in a very important field, which is improving educational competences and counteracting the effects of chronic stress, as well as social exclusion of families who care for children with autism spectrum disorders.

Educational activities are aimed at modifying the child's behavior, which will make it possible to obtain the effect of the student's and therapist's work, acquire the ability to carry out orders, eliminate undesirable disruptive, self-destructive, and aggressive behaviors. This impact zone is also aimed at assimilating the child with educational skills and knowledge necessary for the implementation of compulsory schooling, introducing a general improvement program, and consolidating all acquired skills. Communication interactions are the basis for building the little patient's independence and the possibility of finding his own place in society, as well as the ability to communicate with him, if not verbally, then with the use of alternative methods of communication. Activities in the social sphere should provide care for the child as well as assistance and advice in dealing with official matters, as well as provide social support to the patient's family.

The last group of interactions that should be applied by a facility that specializes in autism spectrum therapy is supportive treatment and physiotherapy. This type of activities is aimed at stimulating development in individual spheres of functioning, improving the tasks of individual senses, their compatibility and integration.

Social integration through therapeutic contact with the animal world and peers as well as occupational therapy also finds its place here. The interaction group based on supportive therapy is an appropriate field for physiotherapists to work with autistic children. In the autism spectrum therapy, the following are used among the physiotherapy departments: manual therapy, hydrotherapy, therapeutic massage, physical therapy, and ergotherapy.

6.2 Neurorehabilitation

It is an important type of individual therapy aimed at intensifying the level of concentration of attention, similar to quantitative indicators in terms of the ratio of beta waves to theta, as well as SMR to theta, as well as in quantitative indicators for functional tests. Neurorehabilitation can be divided into two types of impact:

- magnetostimulation —i.e., the use of slowly changing magnetic fields in the patient in order to influence the bioelectrical activity of the cerebral cortex, especially on such phenomena as: concentration of attention, feeling of physical and mental relaxation, and thus on many other functions and cognitive processes,

- EEG—biofeedback training—that is, work based on a biological feedback system, thanks to which the patient learns to emit brain waves at the frequency imposed on him by the therapist so that his body can be brought into the desired state of activity (concentration of attention, relaxation) [32].

Research shows that systematic EEG biofeedback training can be an effective form of therapy for autistic children in the areas of verbal, physical, and social communication. Scientific research also shows improved speech, balance, understanding, and facial expressions in children with autism. The trainings also turned out to be helpful in reducing sensory sensitivity and in improving the response to changes in the environment. Trainings should be conducted at least once a week. Greater and definitely faster effects of the therapy are obtained by training two or three times a week. The minimum number of trainings to achieve the goal and consolidate the achieved effects of the therapy is about 20 sessions. [33].

6.3 Sensory integration (SI)

Sensory integration is the stimulation of the neurological process so that it organizes the sensations flowing from the body so that they can be used for purposeful action. Sensory integration disorders consist in incorrect processing of stimuli within the sensory, vestibular, visual, auditory, olfactory, and taste systems. The function of the analyzers is correct. They are clinically manifested by increased or decreased sensitivity to stimuli, abnormal levels of attention, poor motor coordination, delayed speech development, and behavioral difficulties. Thanks to AI therapy, the child's brain, after collecting information from all senses, leads to their recognition, segregation, interpretation, and integration with information already possessed in order to be able to prepare an answer in the form of an appropriate motor reaction. The basis for working with this method consists of three basic sensory systems: the surface/tactile sensing system (whose receptors are located on the skin and are responsible for the reception of tactile, pain, and thermal stimuli), the deep/proprioceptive sensing system (with receptors receiving stimuli coming from tendons and muscles), and the vestibular/vestibular system (in which the receptors are located in the inner ear and receive impulses that inform us about the position of the head in relation to the force of gravity). Therapy based on loose and liquid materials—in children with the autism spectrum, it aims to overcome the resistance which, due to their hypersensitivity in the area of superficial sensation, does not want to touch anything, which is wet, rough, slippery, warm, cold, etc., different structure, temperature, texture, or liquidity. Working in the darkroom, it is a method aimed at increasing the level of concentration of attention. Classes are conducted in a darkened room.

Working with an autistic child takes place in three stages:

1. focusing attention on a moving image (e.g., using a projector with thematic dials or liquid colors),

2. work with point and laser light,

3. task projections in ultraviolet light.

6.4 Auditory training

Auditory training using the Tomatis method—it is audio-psycho-linguistic stimulation carried out with the help of a device called the electronic ear. They make up her sessions, which consist in listening to appropriately configured sound material through special headphones, as well as additional consultations together with an audio-psycho-phonological assessment. Through appropriate training, this method allows to achieve good results when the child's listening process is disturbed, i.e., processing and analyzing auditory stimuli through the nervous system. And in the case of hearing disorders, it does not apply, i.e., when the sound reception is incorrect due to organic hearing damage.

6.5 Movement-based therapeutic interventions

Relaxation—it is used during the occurrence of excessive muscle tension or strong psychomotor agitation often occurring in children with the autism spectrum.

The most commonly used relaxation techniques are:

- relaxation based on light and sound—as individual classes conducted on a waterbed in a darkened room, with a delicate play of lights from bubble columns and music from external speakers or mounted in a waterbed (which gives an additional effect in the form of gentle vibrations for the body),
- surface and deep massage—which is a full body massage that stimulates the surface and deep feeling, relaxes the muscles, and eliminates connective tissue adhesions,
- hydrotherapeutic massage—a treatment performed in a hydromassage bathtub,
- aquatherapy—in the form of treatments carried out through fabrics (wraps, wrapping, rubbing, washing),
- aromatic baths,
- pearl baths,
- water therapy—as group activities in a therapeutic pool, the aim of which is not only to achieve relaxation effects, but also to integrate with peers, play together, and learn to follow instructions [32]. Aspects of psychological therapies applied to children with autism spectrum disorders and their families are also taken into account [34].

Therapy using the Knill method—it is a therapy in the form of a session, which is always accompanied by similar rituals (preparing props, adopting similar positions, starting exercises when certain music is turned on, etc.). These types of classes allow you to establish contact with the child, develop its activity in time and space, teach the acquisition of planning and foresight skills, as well as develop hearing and motor coordination.

Sherborne Developmental Movement Method is a system of movement games and exercises, the main task of which is to develop the emotional and social sphere in a child, as well as to develop awareness of himself and other people. Groups of exercises thanks to which you can solve specific problems occurring in people with developmental disorders:

- exercises leading to getting to know your own body;
- exercises that help to gain self-confidence and trust in a partner as well as a sense of security in contact;
- exercises that teach how to establish contact and cooperate in a group. Here we distinguish different types of relational games: caring—"with" together against;

- exercises leading to cooperation in a group;

- creative exercises.

There is no competition-inducing exercise. Children are praised and encouraged to be active. By gaining self-confidence, children are more likely to participate in other forms of therapy [15].

Dennison's method also known as The Brain Gym is a set of exercises aimed at integrating the cerebral hemispheres in order to work more effectively. Dennison's method is teaching with activating methods to turn on the natural mechanisms of mind and body integration through specially organized movements. Through the use of exercise, all parts of the brain turn on and work together to improve each chosen skill. It is a method that improves the effectiveness of learning, communication, creativity, and work efficiency. A very important factor in using this form in working with an autistic person is learning how to relax, relieve tension, and cope with stress.

The method of a good start aims to improve and improve the interaction of motor and psyche in a child through correction as well as compensation of disturbed functions. This method has various aspects, both prophylactic and therapeutic, as well as an equally important diagnostic aspect that allows assessing the type, causes, and depth of dysfunction in a given patient. Scheme of therapeutic work with this method begins with introductory classes, then basic classes (motor, motor-auditory and motor-auditory-visual), and final classes (they are calming, relaxing).

Therapy according to Masgutova's program consists in organizing neurosensory conditions for the proper functioning of schemas that are components of the reflex wheel, and they include the sensory organ, then the processing of the sensory-proprioceptive stimulus, and the motor organ. The techniques of this therapy are focused on re-patterning procedures, i.e., coordinating new relationships between the components of the reflex wheel. The results of reflex integration influence their maturation and the structure of planned and controlled movement. Their task is to improve the functioning of the sensor, motor coordination, and quality of movement. They improve the communication skills, concentration of attention as well as spatial organization.

6.6 Structured improvement

It is a group of activities included in the strictly defined framework of their course. They consist in providing the environment of a child with ASD with permanent structures: physical (including establishing permanent places to play, eat, move, didactic tasks, eliminate disruptive stimuli, no sudden radical changes); visual (visibility of materials and teaching aids, the use of clear, unambiguous pictures, symbols, visual organization of activities and tasks, day plan); visual marking of areas in the room with symbols, pictograms; structures in the form of fixed rules, rules and a fixed schema, e.g., daily schedule.

6.7 Relationship-based therapy

The Relationship Development Intervention (RDI) method is based on work with children performed by parents at home. It consists in providing parents with tools to effectively teach their child the skills that make up dynamic intelligence and increase his motivation to work. It focuses on changing what characterizes autism, i.e., thinking stiffness, reluctance to change, lack of motivation, inability to see someone else's perspective, difficulties in communication. The RDI program was based on working on five basic skills, typical of the so-called dynamic intelligence, necessary for normal functioning in life, which are also the five basic deficits found in people with autism. These are:

- dynamic analysis—the ability to analyze information in terms of what is important at a given moment, what to focus on, setting priorities;
- experience sharing communication—using the so-called declarative speech that does not give ready-made answers, forces you to think, arouses curiosity;
- episodic memory—memory of events and emotions that accompanied the event. The memory necessary to create our personal history and build a sense of competence and motivation;
- flexible thinking—the ability to quickly adapt to the situation, openness to changes, the ability to act under the criterion: "good enough";
- self-awareness—the basic skill to understand that everyone is different and that our interactions and behaviors affect other people. It is also an essential skill to build motivation.

7. Manual techniques (cranial therapy and microkinesitherapy)

They consist in the use of forms of minimal pressure on the patient's body in specific places in order to relieve the remaining tensions and muscle or fascial blockages. In autistic children, the most important thing is to eliminate blockages that are located in the bones of the skull and the entire hyoid system (muscles of the neck, collarbones, skull base, palate, temporomandibular joint).

8. Ergotherapy

Ergotherapy is recognized as one of the branches of physiotherapy and is based mainly on medical, psychological, social, and craft knowledge. It is used in the case of movement, sensory, nerve conduction, and mental disorders in patients of all ages, including older children. Its aim is to restore or acquire mobility, overcome difficulties in performing self-service activities, as well as other activities of everyday life. The consequence of ergotherapy should be for the child to obtain the greatest possible independence, independence, and life activity. Among the ergotherapeutic forms of work used in the treatment of patients affected by the autism spectrum, it is worth mentioning: occupational therapy, creative therapy, art therapy, music therapy, culinary therapy, psychodrama, rock climbing, or therapeutic and recreational tourism.

9. TEACCH

The origins of the TEACCH program go back to the 1970s. Eric Schopler's research resulted in the creation of an unusual, for those times, program of work with autistic people. This program differed from previous methods of work by recognizing the role of the parent as a co-therapist, full involvement of parents in the therapy, which was a stark contrast to the earlier attitude of blaming them for the autism spectrum of the child. The TEACCH program was also a structured program as opposed to the widely used play therapy.

The most important assumption of the TEACCH program is the individualization of the therapy program for each child and the broadly understood cooperation between professional therapists and parents. Parents are treated as an invaluable source of knowledge about their children, they are treated on an equal footing with therapists, the parent and the therapist learn from each other by creating a therapeutic team. Parents bring dedication, commitment, motivation, knowledge of the child to the team, and professionals bring knowledge about professional techniques. PEP-R tools are used to individualize therapy.

The TEACCH program is a comprehensive program, it includes various types of therapy for autistic children, it uses, for example, behavioral therapy or sensory integration and many other programs that will prove effective for a given child. The diagnosis of the TEACCH program is divided into several stages. The first is the initial diagnosis, which is based on the individual assessment of the child by PEP-R, CARS, or AAPEP. With the help of these tools, the predisposition, skills, and potential of the child are established. The obtained results are supplemented with an environmental interview. Then the whole family is included in the program of meetings at the center, which aims to work with both the child and the parent. The child therapist works with the child, learns about its strengths and weaknesses, determines the initial therapy plan, while the family counselor looks after the parents, helps them find their way around the situation, helps them understand the nature of the impairment, and learns from it about the child. Then the therapy program is jointly established. Once this program is approved by the parents, the therapist arranges the exercises to be performed at home.

10. Option method

The option method was developed by a Kaufman couple through experiences with their own autistic child. They were looking for a therapy for their son before an official diagnosis was made. They knew that the earlier the therapy started, the greater the possibilities and chances for the child. They also realized that leaving their son in their own world without trying to understand and help them may result in the deepening of autistic behaviors, the consolidation of autistic patterns, and the resulting emotional problems. Barry Kaufman became interested in the Option Method derived from the Attitude of Options, that is, "To love someone and be happy with him" [35].

This method consisted in revising one's own beliefs, which made a person unhappy. She assumed that you can choose your own beliefs, which affects your feelings and behavior. The starting point for therapy is therefore work with parents, its aim is to teach the parent to accept the child, understand his behavior, and the parent also learns educational techniques. The next stage of therapy is joining the child's activity, imitating his behavior in order to show him that he is next to a presence full of love and approval and that he wants to make contact in a way that is possible for the child. The next stage is motivating the child to want to make contact, to want to go beyond the rigid framework of their behavior. At this stage, it is all the time important to imitate the child and constant presence, stimulate the child with himself, with his closeness, try to establish contact through various types of clever tricks, such as making the child meet with the eyes of the parent. Making eye contact is very important for the child to it acquired awareness of the existence of parents, acquired knowledge about parents so that it could learn through limitation. Eye contact is essential for significant progress to be made.

11. Behavioral interventions

Applied Behavior Analysis (ABA) is a scientific approach to understanding different behaviors. It uses many years of experience, numerous studies, theories, and principles of behavior understood very broadly [36]. SAZ is based on causal (also known as instrumental) conditioning. Behavioral interventions use, inter alia, proactive strategies, i.e., various techniques related to manipulating the stimuli that precede the behavior. The most frequently used of them are: adapting the program to the child's abilities, interweaving difficult and easy tasks, presenting tasks at the right pace, allowing the child to make a choice, adjusting the environment to be the optimal place for learning, and using various types of prompts [36]. Behavior-related interventions are also included in this category, and reinforcement is of particular importance here. Reinforcement can be positive or negative. Positive reinforcement occurs when, after a child becomes involved in a behavior, he or she receives the desired stimulus. It is important to take care of the variety of reinforcements and to individualize them so as not to become saturated with them. These can be the child's favorite treats, the therapist's attention, attractive toys, or pleasant activity with the therapist. The second type of reinforcement, negative reinforcement, occurs when the child's involvement in a given behavior causes the unwanted stimulus to be withdrawn. A particular type of enhancement is differential enhancement, where desired behaviors are enhanced and undesirable behaviors are suppressed. This results in the reduction of many undesirable behaviors of the child and teaching functional and desired responses in a given situation.

12. Modeling

Modeling is an effective way to teach a child how to do something by showing him or her. Children can learn a lot by observing and imitating the behavior of their parents, siblings, peers, and teachers. We distinguish between two types of modeling: "live" and video-modeling. The first type is that the therapist (model) presents a certain behavior to imitate and the child repeats it. It is important that the behavior to be imitated is well described and that each of the modelers presents it to the child in the same way. During modeling, the child should be focused in order to be able to observe the model's behavior well. In the final stage, a method of withdrawing modeling should be developed so that the learned behavior occurs spontaneously and in appropriate situations without the participation of the model. The second type, video modeling, is where a certain behavior is prerecorded and the child imitates the behavior observed in the video [37].

13. Methods of supporting communication

Various forms of assisted communication are used in autistic children. The term *Alternative and Supportive Methods of Communication* (AAC) groups methods that enable people with speech disabilities to communicate with their environment.

13.1 Makaton

The Makaton method is one of many alternative communication tools. It uses signs, i.e., gestures and symbols. Gestures and symbols can be used along with speech, then they have an auxiliary function, reinforcing the message, or in the case of lack of speech they constitute an independent method of communication. Graphic symbols are used with Makaton's gestures. They are black and white, simple pictures that accurately reflect the concepts they represent. The basic vocabulary includes 450 symbols and approximately 7,000,000 supplementary symbols. Each country has its own set of graphic symbols. The Makaton program was originally developed in the United Kingdom by Margaret Walker, a speech therapist and psychiatrist. The Polish version of Makaton was developed by Bogusława Kaczmarek. The changes included both gestures and graphic symbols. The basic vocabulary is 350 words very similar in all countries in Europe, in addition, in Poland, 100 words characteristic of our culture or customs. It is also emphasized that the applied therapeutic methods are carried out under additional aggravating conditions of Covid-19 [38].

Makaton Program users can be children and adults with different communication disorders profiles. The use of the language of symbols and gestures does not pose a threat to the development of speech as speech is used together with symbols or gestures whenever possible, and when it develops on a level sufficient for communication, the language of signs and symbols is discontinued [39].

13.2 Therapeutic process in the event of a pandemic

The first case of the SARS-CoV-2 virus in Poland was recorded on March 4, 2020, and less than a week later, the World Health Organization granted COVID-19 pandemic status, which resulted in changes in the functioning of families around the world. People with autism as people with disabilities were included in the group at high risk of contracting the virus. A number of changes concerned not only education, but also care and rehabilitation [40].

When on March 11, the work of educational system institutions was limited, it was also associated with the closure of educational and upbringing institutions, special schools, as well as specialized training and revalidation and upbringing centers [41]. Even in the first half of March, some support centers were also closed, and the children had to stay at home, without specialist care, which certainly made it difficult functioning of the family and initiated the growing problems of parents [40]. Due to the fact that families with children were locked at home, it was extremely important that the child continued to develop properly and make progress despite the lack of treatment with a specialist. One of the examples of replacing sensory therapy is sensory-motor games that stimulate the senses and reduce irritability in a child:

1. creating a harp from a box of chocolates and recipe rubber bands—the child chooses the number of rubber bands on his own and puts them on the boxes, then he can pluck them like strings while humming his favorite songs, while the

parent can help "tune the strings" by stretching or loosening the rubber bands in order to spend others sounds, this game affects touch, sight, and hearing,

2. "Jump cushion"—stacking all kinds of pillows, quilts, and other soft materials in a pile, preferably in the middle of the room, providing space around the top of the pillows, the child will be able to jump while plunging into a soft pile, this game exerts pressure on muscles and joints as well as tactile stimuli and proprioceptive,

3. hug combined with rolling—a game affecting the vestibular system and tactile stimuli, consisting in placing the child on the stomach of an adult lying on his back in a hug and slowly rolling over the couch or other soft surfaces,

4. "Listen and draw" – a game involving playing music and conveying emotions related to the sounds heard by the child by drawing, preferably using crayons in a standing or lying position, the game strengthens the receptors of hearing, sight, and touch,

5. "Hammer and nails" – admittedly, a game for larger children that develops hand coordination, visual skills and spatial orientation, consisting in hammering small nails into a piece of wood by the child, but it can be replaced by hammering a golf ball into, for example, polystyrene or other soft material.

These sensory games not only help children to cope with stress and isolation, but can also be used at home as an addition to sensory therapy classes [41]. An important aspect is to create an environment for the child to facilitate sensory processing. For a child with autism, the highest priority is a safe environment that makes it easier for them to focus. Parents should adapt the environment in which the child is to be with other household members on a continuous basis to his needs. The level of the child's arousal depends on his environment. Any loud sounds should be eliminated by introducing soft background music, providing subdued colors and natural lighting, as well as organizing each room and clearly defining the passages. The apartment should be warm, but not too hot, and the smells should be subdued and controlled (no use or limitation of perfumes, disinfectants, cleaning products) [41].

Kashman and Mora created in their essay a sensory cheat sheet for the sense of touch, proprioceptive, and vestibular. And so, the sense of touch is best influenced by loose products such as rice or dry beans, modeling clay, or a massage with a balm. The sense of proprioception is influenced by e.g., walking, even in place, stomping, placing food cans (with a load). On the other hand, races, jumping on the floor or playing with a scarf are good examples of games that affect the vestibular sense [28].

Karen Simmons, based on a short sentence spoken by her friend: "Fear may be the most destructive and harmful virus known to mankind." SARS-CoV-2 virus. These are:

1. "The essence of our being is love,

2. Health is inner peace, healing is Letting go of fear,

3. Giving and taking are the same

4. We can let go of the past and the future

5. Only now counts, every moment is dedicated to giving

6. We can learn to love ourselves and others by forgiving, not judging

7. We can become seekers of love, not seekers of wine

8. We can choose and focus on keeping our inner peace no matter what happens outside,

9. We are students and teachers for each other,

10. We can focus on all of life, not just parts of it,

11. Since love is Eternal, death need not be seen as something terrible

12. We can always see others as loving or fearful and extend the cry for help in love." [41]

These so-called positive attitudes principles were intended to help, in these extremely difficult times, especially for parents to remain calm and pass it on to a child with autism spectrum disorder [41].

14. Discussion

Progress in research on the autism spectrum and its genesis results in more and more forms of development support therapy. However, since the causes of the autism spectrum disorder have not been clearly identified, there is no "cure" for the disorder. Educational, behavioral, and rehabilitation influences play the most important role in the treatment of autism. Therapy should be comprehensive and carried out in specialized centers. The nervous system is so plastic that when properly stimulated, it can make up for many deficits. The sooner a child is cared for, the better the results. Currently, there are many forms of therapy available to improve the functioning of an autistic child. Autism is not a fully curable disorder, but with the use of appropriate therapeutic programs, some people are able to achieve such an improvement that they can function independently.

Children with autism spectrum disorder (ASD) are less likely to participate in physical activity than their age-related peers, and it has been suggested that physical therapists (PT) have the potential to facilitate their participation. Currently, no study has investigated the potential role of PT in increasing participation in physical activity (PA). The purpose of this qualitative study was to investigate the experiences of PT and the outlook for working with children with ASD and to explore potential directions in which PT could potentially increase PA. Methods: Ten pediatric PTs in Canada were interviewed and the data analyzed by thematic analysis. Results: Three themes were identified: the role of PT, perceived lack of expertise, trust and training, and structural and systemic barriers. The accounts emphasize the social and institutional complexity and limitations of PT's potential promotion of PA in children with ASD. Participants supported primarily a consultative role whereby physical therapists can educate themselves and collaborate with parents, teachers, and social service providers to improve gross motor development and individualize PA needs. Conclusions: These results indicate how PT may be involved in enhancing PA in children with ASD [7].

Stasolla, Boccasini, and Perilli (2017) presented a literature review on assistive technology-based programs supporting the adaptive behavior of children with autism spectrum disorders that are broadly understood and designed to bridge the gap between human/individual abilities and/or skills and requests for environment. In particular, AT builds a link that enables people with ASD to gain independence and self-determination. By using the AT configuration, individuals with ASD may be able to achieve an active role, positive participation, beneficial occupation, and/or performance of functional daily activities. Moreover, they could be enabled to improve their social image, attractiveness, and status, while reducing the burden on families and carers. In short, people with ASD would cope positively with their environment. At least two functional goals can be achieved through an AT-based intervention, namely (a) evaluation and (b) recovery. In the case of the autism spectrum, El Kaliouby and Robinson (2007, p. 3) indicated that assistive technologies can be "divided into two broad categories," i.e. therapeutic and prosthetic, with therapeutic technologies aimed at helping people cope with disabilities or specific deficiencies through curricula and interventions [42].

The review of the abovementioned methods of therapy for people with ASD shows that there is no one method that would cover all the needs of a child with ASD and his family. It seems appropriate to select therapies and working methods in accordance with the child's needs and based on his strengths.

The latest research (not published: E.Trylinska-Tekielska The sense of empathy and the sense of stress in the group of parents of children from the autism spectrum in the pandemic period, 2022) shows that the personality traits of the closest relatives are a very important rehabilitation factor for children from the autism spectrum disorder. The child's caregivers show the greater stress they experience, certainly a very important factor in preparing the child to function in society. It is also important that the society understands and respects the child's needs from the autism spectrum.

15. Conclusion

The assessment of the social functioning of a person with an autism spectrum disorder is in contradiction with the dominant image of the autism spectrum as an ailment that disrupts functioning in the social sphere.

Most people believe that an autistic person is capable of making friends, working professionally, and living independently; the general public believes that a person with ASD is able to start a family. At the same time, the dominant opinion is that a child with spectrum autism is not able to cope in an ordinary school.

Behind this contradiction may be the belief that autism is a predominantly childhood condition, out of which to some extent "outgrows," and an adult on the spectrum copes better in society than a child.

The problems of families of children with the autism spectrum have remained unchanged for years: it is primarily the lack of professional help in childcare, social exclusion, lack of emotional support, lack of knowledge about the autism spectrum, and lack of funds for living.

A specialist or a group of specialists should work with the child, who will first of all give the correct diagnosis and repeat it, tracking the child's development and adjusting the therapy to the changes in the child's behavior and its health condition.

People with the autism spectrum disorder during the pandemic reported experiencing higher than usual anxiety, nervousness, and tension, as well as anger.

A very small group of people on the autism spectrum have benefited from therapeutic support for the pandemic; most people did not receive any form of therapy.

Due to the fact that families with children were locked at home, it was extremely important that the child continued to develop properly and make progress despite the lack of treatment with a specialist.

The entire burden of carrying out therapy rested with families.

The crumbs of autism reside in each of us.

Author details

Elzbieta Trylinska-Tekielska*, Dorota Pietraszewska, Iwona Stanisawska and Ada Holak
College of Rehabilitation, Warsaw, Poland

*Address all correspondence to: etek@poczta.onet.pl

IntechOpen

© 2022 The Author(s). Licensee IntechOpen. This chapter is distributed under the terms of the Creative Commons Attribution License (http://creativecommons.org/licenses/by/3.0), which permits unrestricted use, distribution, and reproduction in any medium, provided the original work is properly cited. (cc) BY

References

[1] Diagnosis-Foundation Help Autism. Available at : https://www.pomocautyzm.org/icd-11-autyzm [01-04-2022]

[2] Wing L, Gould J. Severe impairments of social interaction and associated abnormalities in children: Epidemiology and classification. Journal of Autism Development Disorders. 1979;**9**:11-29

[3] Rutkiewicz D. "Own Program" Therapy and Rehabilitation of Children with the Autism Spectrum. 2019

[4] Hoffman JE. Clinical symptoms and diagnosis of autism and other pervasive developmental disorders. Psychiatry after Diploma. 2009;**6**:45-54

[5] Yates K. Autism diagnosis. Medical Practise Pediatrician. 2009;**3**:79-88

[6] Komender J, Jagielska G, Bryńska A. Autism and Asperger 's Syndrome. Warsaw: Medical Publishing House; 2009

[7] Campos C , Duck M, McQuillan R, Brazill L, Malik S. Exploring the Role of Physiotherapists in the Care of Children with Autism Spectrum

[8] Rybakowski F, Białek A, Chojnicka E, Dziechciarz P, Horvath A, Janas-Kozik M, et al. Autism spectrum disorders - epidemiology, symptoms, comorbidity and diagnosis. Polish Psychiatry. 2014;**4**:653-665

[9] Chojnicka I, Płoski R. Polish version of the interview for diagnosing the autism spectrum ADI-R. Psychiatria Polska. 2012;**2**:249-259

[10] Pisula E. A small child with an autism spectrum. Diagnosis and Therapy, Gdańskie Wydawnictwo Psychologiczne, Sopot. 2005, 36-88.

[11] Pietras T, Witusik A, Gałecki P. Autism Spectrum – Epidemiology, Diagnosis and Therapy. Wrocław: Continuo; 2010. pp. 18-199

[12] Schopler E, Reichler RJ, Bashford A, Lansing MD, Marcus LM. Individualized Ocean Therapy and Therapy for Autistic Children and Children with Developmental Disorders. Gdańsk: Association for Help for Autistic People; 1995. pp. 17-19

[13] Tuchman R, Rapin I. Epilepsy in autism. Lancet Neurology. 2002;**1**:352-358

[14] Sherborne W. Movement Developing. Warsaw: PWN; 2012. pp. 7-49

[15] Lewartowska L. Spectrum of Childhood Autism: Issues of Diagnosis and Therapy Krakow. Oficyna Wydawnicza Impuls; 2005. pp. 27-123

[16] Grrhan A, Olajossy M. Olajossy-Hilkesberger L (Neuroanatomical, genetic and neurochemical aspects of the spectrum of childhood autism). Psychiatric. 2013;**47**(6):1101-1111

[17] Dworzańska E, Makarewicz A, Koncewicz R, Hołowicka-Kłapeć P, Mitosek-Szewczyk K. Neurological Disorders in Autism, Health and Well-being. 1/2015. pp. 38-44

[18] Warren F. The Society That Kills Your Children: The Autistic Child and Its Parents, Educational Guide. red T Gałkowski, Warsaw, PTWzK. 1984. pp. 19-38

[19] Lange K, Tarnowska E, Krusiec J, Gruczy E, Kowalska D, Kozłowska M.

Influence of nutrition of children with spectrum disorders autism on selected eating behavior children with autism spectrum disorders on selected dieters behavior. Problems in High Epidemiology. 2018;**99**(1):12-20

[20] Randolph-Gips M, Srinivasan P. Modeling autism: A systems biology approach. Journal of Clinical Bioinforma. 2012;**2**(1):17

[21] Whiteley P, Haracopos D, Knivsberg AM, et al. The ScanBrit randomized , controlled, single-blind study of and gluten- and casein-free dietary intervention for children with autism spectrum disorders. Nutritional Neuroscience. 2010;**13**(2):87-100

[22] Pennesi CM, Klein LC. Effectiveness of the gluten-free, casein-free diets for children diagnosed with autism spectrum disorder: Based on parental report. Nutritional Neurosciences. 2012;**15**(2):85-91

[23] Krigsman A, Boris M, Goldblatt A, Stott C. Clinical presentation and histologic findings at ileocolonoscopy in children with Autistic Spectrum Disorder and Chronic Gastrointestinal Symptoms. Autism Insights. 2010;**2**:1-11

[24] De Magistris L, Familiari V, Pascotto A, et al. Alterations of the intestinal barrier in patients with Autism Spectrum Disorders and in their first-degree relatives. Journal of Pediatric Gastroenterology Nutrition. 2010;**51**(4):418-424

[25] Modabbernia A, Velthorst E, Reichenberg A. Environmental risk factors for autism: An evidence-based review of systematic reviews and meta-analyzes. Mothly Autism. 2017;**8**:13

[26] Jarosz M, Brajbisz M, Sanicka A. Nutritional treatment of autism - opportunities and threats. Nutrition | Human and Metabolism. 2015;**XLIII**(3):176-188

[27] Jarosz M, Bribisz M. Nutrition in the prevention of autism. Human Nutrition and Metabolism. 2015;**XLIII**(2):34-46

[28] Zalewska A, Pawłowicz K, Cezary Roman C. Disorders in the development of communication in children with autism spectrum disorders. In: Kulak E, Łukaszczuk C, Lewko J, Kulak W, editors. The Holistic Dimension of Contemporary Medicine Białystok, Medical University of Białystok. 2021;(8):685-695

[29] Grad D. Parents as Invaluable Therapists of Their Own Children with Disabilities in the Field of Early Development Support. In: Palak Z, Wójcik M, editors. Pedagogical therapy for children with special developmental and educational needs. New Faces of Therapy in Special Education. Lublin: UMCS; 2016. pp. 73-87

[30] Pisula E. Family in the Treatment of a Child with Autism. APS 2003 edition. Warsaw. p. 117

[31] Pisula E. A Small Child with Autism. Sopot GWP; 2005. pp. 36-88

[32] Kuliński W, Orlik T, Zeman K. Physiotherapy in pediatry Warsaw. PZWL. 2012. pp. 165-173

[33] Available from: http://autyzm.org.pl/terapie-wspomagajace/biofeedback-w-autyzmiev [01-04-2022]

[34] Trylińska-Tekielska E. Psychologist at the Hospice Warsaw Scholar. 2015

[35] Kaufmann BN. The Awakening of Our Son. Warsaw: Synapsis Foundation; 1994. pp. 30-79

[36] Suchowierska M, Ostaszewski P, Bąbel P. Terapia behawioralna dzieci z autyzmem GWP. Sopot. 2015

[37] Findings and Conclusions: National Standards Project, Phase 2. Addressing the Need for Evidence-BasedPractice Guidelines for Autism Spectrum Disorders. 2015

[38] Trylinska-Tekielska E. Working in a hospice - predictors of starting work in a hospice and their consequences in the group of professional workers, hospice volunteers and ordinary volunteers - Psychological Model of the Team working in the conditions of the exhibition. SilvaRerum Poznań. 2019

[39] Komunikacja alternatywna. Available from: MAKATON - język gestów i symboli jako Program Rozwoju Komunikacji dostępne pod adresem www.makaton.pl [01=04-2022]

[40] Macałka E, Nieradka F, Beginning G. COVID-19 and autism spectrum disorders. Selected strategies of supporting people with ASD during a pandemic, Studia Psychologica XIII. 2020

[41] Regulation of the Minister of National Education of 11 March 2020 on the temporary limitation of the functioning of education system units in connection with preventing, counteracting and combating COVID-19, Journal of Laws. 2020. Item 410

[42] Goosen L. Spectrum disorders Autism Assistive Technologies for Children and Adolescents. DOI: 10.4018/978-1-7998-7430-0